Yoga and Ayurveda

Self-Healing and Self-Realization

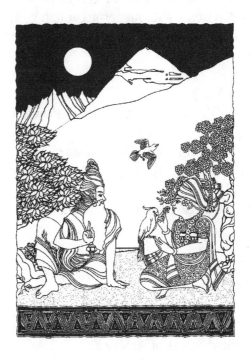

By David Frawley

LOTUS

DISCLAIMER

EDITOR: Parvati Markus
COVER & PAGE DESIGN/LAYOUT: Paul Bond, Art & Soul Design
COVER ILLUSTRATION: Dee Davis
ILLUSTRATIONS: Georg Feurstein (nadis), Margo Gal (spiritual heart, prana and asana drawings), Kent Lew (chakras), Hinduism Today (yogi as fire)
BACK COVER PHOTO: Mira Foung

First Edition, 1999
Reprinted, 2009

Printed in the United States of America

Library of Congress Cataloging-in-Publication-Data
Yoga and Ayurveda. Self-Healing and Self-Realization
includes bibliographical references.
ISBN: 978-0-9149-5581-8   98-75820
                                                          CIP

Published by:
Lotus Press, P.O. Box 325, Twin Lakes, Wisconsin 53181
web: www.lotuspress.com
e-mail: lotuspress@lotuspress.com
800-824-6396

Table of Contents

Foreword

I have come to think of my friend David Frawley as a Hindu pundit in a Western body. This is well captured by his spiritual name Vamadeva Shastri. In Sanskrit, a shastrin (nominative shastri) is a person learned in the shastras, the scholastic textbooks. David Frawley's entire thinking and life revolve around Indic culture and spirituality, and whenever I ask him any question about Yoga, Ayurveda, or the Vedas, his knowledge (vijnana) and wisdom (jnana) invariably bubble forth like a refreshing spring. Since the early 1980s, he has made his insights into India's magnificent spiritual and medical traditions available to Western students through a series of publications.

This new book highlights the close connection between Yoga and Ayurveda, both of which are fundamental holistic disciplines. They intersect in the concept of somatic and psychospiritual wholeness. Yoga focuses on spiritual integration through self-transcendence culminating in Self-realization. Ayurveda focuses on psychosomatic integration through comprehensive health care culminating in openness to self-transcendence and Self-realization.

One of the hallmarks of Yoga is balance, and thus practitioners of this ancient art and science must pay proper attention to both the body and the mind. Sometimes over-zealous Yoga enthusiasts seek to cultivate meditation and higher states of consciousness apart from the physical body, but the body is the ground for realizing enlightenment. If we don't take care of the body, it is likely to succumb to illness sooner or later. Remember, we all have our karmas (read: genetic program and external life situations) to contend with! In Yoga, illness is considered one of the obstacles to successful completion of the yogic process. If you question this, try meditating with a toothache or while feeling sick to your stomach. It can be done, of course, but it presupposes considerable skill in concentration. Somatic imbalances readily give rise to mental disturbances, and vice versa. Therefore, cultivating a trong, healthy body and training the mind should go hand in hand, and both pursuits should ideally be powered by a desire for Self-realization.

Both Yoga and Ayurveda are enjoying immense popularity in the West at the moment. But both disciplines are also subject to considerable distortion. David Frawley's new book could not have been more timely. It offers a most valuable overview of the connecting points between Yoga and Ayurveda and shows how both disciplines are relevant to contemporary spiritual practice.

In particular, this book contains many helpful practical pointers, which will help you to understand your constitutional type in Ayurvedic terms. This, in turn, will assist you in choosing the right kind of yogic postural or meditation practice. The yogic path is intrinsically challenging, and wise practitioners welcome any information that will benefit them even a little bit. Thus the typological knowledge of Ayurveda is one of the best-kept secrets of Yoga. If you make little progress on the yogic path, it is perhaps because you are on the wrong track. Understanding your constitutional type is important not only when determining your diet or a course of medical treatment but also when embarking on spiritual practice. All tracks are equally good and serviceable, but you must have the right axle width to fit on a given track and reach your destination smoothly and safely, or at all. If you have arrived at the understanding that life is a pilgrimage that ends (or really begins) with enlightenment or liberation (moksha), then you will find this book to be an indispensable guide.

Georg Feuerstein, Ph.D., Director, Yoga Research Center

Author of *The Shambhala Encyclopedia of Yoga*,
The Shamballa Guide to Yoga, Tantra: The Path of Ecstasy, etc.

Preface

Yoga and Ayurveda are two closely related spiritual or sacred sciences rooted in the Vedic tradition of India. Ayurveda is the Vedic science of healing for both body and mind. Yoga is the Vedic science of Self-realization that depends upon a well-functioning body and mind. Both disciplines developed together and have always been used together. Therefore, those who are interested in one would benefit from studying the other. However, most books on yoga in the West speak little of Ayurveda. Though all ayurvedic books speak of yoga, so far there has been no single book on Ayurveda and yoga published in the West; hence the need of the present publication.

Yoga and Ayurveda are far more than physical exercise or bodily healing systems such as we tend to view them today, however important these aspects may be. Both classical yoga and Ayurveda look to the whole human being, which is not only body, but mind and soul. Both address all our needs — from physical health and well-being to the unfoldment of our higher consciousness. Therefore, I have oriented this book to the broader view that could be called "integral yoga" and "integral Ayurveda." This is traditionally called *pancha kosha* yoga and *pancha kosha* Ayurveda, meaning yoga and Ayurveda of the five sheaths, which refers to the physical body, *prana*, mind, intelligence, and soul as well as our higher Self. It is also defined as yoga and Ayurveda of the three bodies (physical, astral and causal) or body, mind and soul.

Yoga and Ayurveda addresses our entire nature, our greater life as a spiritual and cosmic being. It examines the broader scope of Ayurveda, which includes not only physical health but also mental health and preparation for the spiritual life. Similarly it looks into the entire field of yoga, the science of *raja yoga* and its eight limbs, from asana to meditation. While the present book does examine the subject of *asana* in one major chapter, a more thorough investigation of the topic is planned as a separate book on Ayurveda and asana.

The book is meant for those who want to explore a deeper level of knowledge than what is usually described in introductory books on these subjects, which are commonly available. It discusses many details about the subtle and causal bodies and their energetics, including much information not previously in print in English. This includes topics such as the seven *agnis*, the three vital essences of *prana, tejas* and *ojas*, the *nadis* and *chakras*, as well as practical methods to unfold these energies. It puts much emphasis on the five *pranas* because prana (the life-force) is the main link between yoga and Ayurveda.

The present book is designed to complement my last book in this field, *Ayurveda and the Mind*, which deals with the psychological aspects and the view of the mind in yoga and Ayurveda. *Ayurveda and the Mind* contains relevant information on mantra and other yogic practices that is not repeated in the present volume and is helpful for those who want more information in these areas. *Yoga and Ayurveda* also interfaces with *Tantric Yoga and the Wisdom Goddesses: Spiritual Secrets of Ayurveda*, which provides additional information on the subtle body and deity worship. My other books on Ayurveda — *Ayurvedic Healing* and the *Yoga of Herbs* (with Dr. Vasant Lad) — deal more with the outer and physical aspects of Ayurveda but refer to yoga in places as well.

Yoga and Ayurveda is divided into three sections:

1. The first section provides the background of Ayurveda and yoga along with their related cosmological principles and

world views, including an understanding of the *doshas* and *gunas*.

2. The second section examines the energetics of the two systems, emphasizing the subtle body and prana, including *kundalini*, the chakras and nadis.

3. The third section shows their common practices from diet and herbs to asana, *pranayama*, mantra and meditation, which enables us to apply the information given in the previous sections.

Like my previous books, the present volume derives much from unpublished writings of Ganapati Muni, chief disciple of Ramana Maharshi, and a great yogi and Ayurvedic teacher as well. These works, passed on to me by Ganapati's disciple, K. Natesan, have proved invaluable in unfolding the yogic secrets of the *Vedas*. The book also relies significantly on the works of Swami Yogeshwarananda. Several chapters derive from articles originally published in the excellent yoga magazine *Yoga International*, including those on *pratyahara*, prana, tejas and ojas, and the chakras.

I would like to thank the various people who have helped me with the book. Sandra Kozak was instrumental in the chapter on asana and is working with me further to develop an Ayurvedic understanding of asana practice that we hope to present in a future volume. Nicholai Bachman produced the charts and the Sanskrit pronunciation guide in the appendix. Gary Kraftsow and Margo Gal offered helpful suggestions relative to asana and pranayama, as did Amadea Morningstar relative to diet. Rudolph Ballantine provided a number of helpful suggestions about the style of the book. Lenny Blank's comments and suggestions were also important.

I would like to dedicate the book to my main teacher not only of Ayurveda but of *dharma*, Dr. B. L. Vashta of Mumbai and Pune, India (1919-1997), a great Ayurvedic doctor, formulator of Ayurvedic products, writer and journalist who for over ten years guided my work and study.

Dr. David Frawley
(Vamadeva Shastri)
Santa Fe, NM
October, 1998

we can live in harmony with the greater universe, not evolving only for ourselves but bringing benefit to all creatures. Ayurveda contains the secrets not only for healing the individual but also for uplifting society, all creatures and the planet itself.

Yoga and Ayurveda are sister sciences that developed together and repeatedly influenced each other throughout history. They are integral parts of the great system of Vedic knowledge which states that all the universe is One Self and that the key to cosmic knowledge lies within our own minds and hearts. As Vedic disciplines, yoga and Ayurveda work together to enhance their great benefits on all levels. They can be integrated with related Vedic or yogic sciences of astrology, architecture, music and language for an even broader approach.[1]

Yoga is first and foremost a science of Self-realization. Its concern is spiritual practice, mainly through meditation, to take us beyond the sorrow and ignorance of the world. It teaches us how to move from our outer bodily and ego-bound identity to our immortal Self that dwells within the heart. Yoga provides the key to all spiritual development, which in the Vedic sense is gaining knowledge of our true nature beyond time, space, death and suffering

Ayurveda is primarily a science of Self-healing aimed at relieving the diseases of body and mind. This does not mean that Ayurveda is merely a method of personal healing which doesn't require help from therapists or doctors. In fact, Ayurveda says that medical practitioners are indispensable in dealing with the complexities of disease and the variabilities of health requirements. Ayurveda as Self-healing means that it is concerned with restoring wholeness, with our inner Self as its ultimate goal, which is spiritual healing.

Ayurveda's concern is alleviating both bodily and mental diseases and promoting both physical and psychological well-being. Yet the ultimate goal of classical Ayurveda, like classical yoga, is Self-realization - the highest form of Self-healing. Ayurveda shows us how to attain optimal health not for outer enjoyment but to provide a wholesome foundation and sufficient energy to pursue the yogic quest.

The link between yoga and Ayurveda is prana, or the life-force. Yoga is the intelligence of prana seeking greater evolutionary transformations, while Ayurveda is its healing power, seeking to consolidate the life-systems it has already developed.

Together, Ayurveda and yoga afford a complete discipline, one which can transform our existence from the physical to the deepest spiritual levels of our being with extraordinary vitality and creativity on all levels.

Yoga and Ayurveda in the West

Yoga is a common term in the Western world today, where yoga classes can be found in every city or neighborhood. Most people identify yoga with the physical postures or asanas that are the most evident side of the system. While yoga asanas can afford a good doorway into the vast temple of yoga, they are hardly the entire structure or its central deity. Eventually, most who look into yoga will come into contact with its broader and more spiritual practices, such as mantra and meditation.

Ayurveda is similarly becoming known in the West today as a special system of natural medicine. There are ayurvedic centers in most cities in the country. Ayurvedic herbs can be found at most health food stores. The idea of ayurvedic constitutional types has been presented in a number of popular books and magazines. However, the physical side of ayurvedic healing through diet and herbs is only part of the system. Its inner aspect, healing the subtle body and the mind (which includes yogic practices and meditation), is the other and perhaps more important half.

A number of yoga centers offer ayurvedic therapies and the two sciences are generally studied together. However, many people who have been introduced to yoga from a physical model may not be fully aware of the importance of its ayurvedic connection. This may include various yoga teachers and yoga therapists, who may themselves have no ayurvedic training.

Traditionally, in India, yoga dealt with the spiritual side of life, what we have introduced as the path of Self-realization. Ayurveda, on the other hand, dealt with both physical and mental disease as well as with the prescription of lifestyle regimens. Yoga as therapy or exercise was traditionally prescribed in an ayurvedic context. Classical yoga therapy was ayurvedic both in theory and in application. This fact should be borne in mind by those using yoga today for healing purposes. They should not ignore the potential benefits of adding ayurvedic insights to yoga therapy. They should learn to understand the ayurvedic effects of yogic practices and not merely try to define yogic healing in terms of modern medicine or modern psychology alone.

The combined study of yoga and Ayurveda is of great importance for each discipline and for helping us understand the whole of life that both sciences address in such a profound manner. Restoring wholeness in body, mind and spirit is what we are all seeking, both individually and collectively.

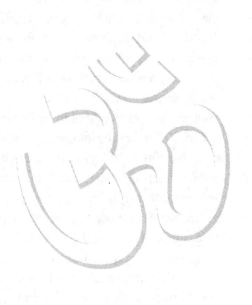

2

Dharma and Tattva

The Universal Philosophy
of Yoga and Ayurveda

Laud the Fire, the seer,
the truth of the Dharma in the sacred rite.
The immortal Fire serves the Gods,
so the Eternal Dharmas are not violated.

RIG VEDA I.12.7; III.3.1

The Way of Dharma

All the great spiritual and healing traditions of the Indian subcontinent are based upon the concept of dharma or natural law. *Dharma* is a Sanskrit word that refers to the laws of truth that govern the universe. Dharma is that which upholds things, a fundamental principle, and literally a pillar. Dharmas are the underlying principles that keep all things in harmony and sustain their higher growth and development. Such dharmic principles, like physical laws, must be the same for all beings. Dharma indicates the foundation of universal law on which we must base our actions for them to gain the support of the universe. Hinduism calls itself *Sanatana Dharma*, or the Eternal Dharma, suggesting a tradition of natural law not limited by time, space or person. Buddhism calls itself *Buddha Dharma*, the natural way of enlightenment.

9

Yoga can be called dharmic spiritual practice, *Yoga Dharma*. Yoga is a dharmic approach to the spiritual life, which is the way of Self-realization. It instructs us to follow our higher dharma, which is to give up outer seeking and strive to know our true nature. All the methodologies of yoga are dharmic in nature, helping us harness natural law and the spiritual forces in nature to transform our consciousness from ignorance to enlightenment.

Ayurveda can be called dharmic medicine. Ayurveda represents a dharmic approach to health and everyday living — natural healing based upon natural law, conscious healing following the laws of consciousness. Ayurveda is the science of health based upon dharmic principles, which seeks to uphold the dharma both in treatment and in its lifestyle regimens. Dharmic living gives us health and happiness, putting us in contact with cosmic forces of beneficence. *Adharmic* living, life contrary to dharma, brings pain and disharmony to all. A dharmic life is the basis of all ayurvedic treatment and all ayurvedic lifestyle regimens. Most psychological problems and emotional disorders are rooted in adharmic living, living out of harmony with the universe. Most physical diseases are based on it as well.

The most important dharmic law is the law of *karma*: as we act, so must we experience the fruit of our actions, not only in this life but in future lives as well. There is an absolute justice in the universe, but this occurs through many incarnations and cannot be seen by a momentary look at human affairs. It is not a justice of outer rewards and punishments but one of the development of consciousness. Dharmic action provides inner peace and happiness and allows us to pursue spiritual practice. Adharmic action constricts our consciousness and consigns us to darkness and turbulence of mind, though it may give us transient external gains.

The most important ethical dharma, sometimes called the supreme dharma, is *ahimsa*, often translated as "non-violence."

More accurately it means "non-harming," having an attitude of mind that does not wish injury to any creature, not merely for human beings, but for plants, animals and the entire natural order. For it to be complete, ahimsa must extend not only to action but also to speech and to thought.

Ahimsa is the most important observance in the practice of yoga and the basis for mental peace, which is not possible if we harbor thoughts of harm for others. How can we sincerely engage in spiritual practices if we are engaged in actions that are violent, destructive, deceptive or manipulative? Ahimsa is the basis of the ayurvedic approach to health and the support of all real healing. Health and well-being arise from a state of mind and a lifestyle that does not project harm onto other creatures.

Ahimsa is behind the ayurvedic recommendation of a vegetarian diet, but it extends to all ayurvedic healing prescriptions. Food should not be based upon cruelty. Food, after all, is a means of providing nourishment. What kind of nourishment can be derived from food that reflects not the energy of love but that of exploitation? Our occupation or vocation in life should also follow an energy of love and not be harmful to other creatures. Unfortunately, modern culture is built upon competition and wasteful consumption in which there is great harm not only to other creatures but to the planet itself.

Above all, medicines should be not be based upon cruelty. Modern medicine believes that by causing harm to other creatures, as in animal testing, we can gain benefits for healing people. Ayurveda states that this is a false logic. We cannot alleviate suffering for one creature by causing suffering to another more helpless. Suffering begets suffering. On the contrary, caring for other creatures benefits our own health, even if it means placing the greater good of all creatures above the good of our own particular species. We cannot triumph in life or wisdom at the expense of the world in which we live.

Ahimsa is the main principle of mental health because it removes the basis for negative emotions to flourish in the mind. It is the main principle of social health because it cuts off the root of social conflict, which is violence stemming from hatred, anger and resentment. Ahimsa, however, is not simply passivity or resignation. Sometimes we must act in a strong or decisive way to prevent harm from occurring, as in the action of a true warrior and defender of dharma. To protect others is another aspect of ahimsa, not often properly understood. It is the basis of the *Kshatriya Dharma*, the Vedic way of the warrior or heroic spirit. For this reason Ayurveda accepts strong therapies, like radical detoxification measures (*Pancha Karma*) to eliminate disease-causing factors, or surgery to protect the life of a person.

Both yoga and Ayurveda teach that we should pray or chant daily universal prayers for peace that project this power of non-violence and its great healing energy.

May all beings find happiness.
May all be free of disease.
May all see what is auspicious.
May no one suffer.
OM, peace, peace, peace.

Ayurveda shares the dharmic principles of yoga, the *yamas* and *niyamas*, which are important principles of right living, that we will discuss under the Paths of Yoga. In addition to universal dharmas, each individual has his or her own personal dharma, or *svadharma*, the law of our own particular nature that shows us our special role and purpose in life. Yoga requires that we find the appropriate dharmic spiritual path and understand our place in the universal unfoldment of consciousness. Ayurveda states that health depends upon discovering our individual dharma and living in harmony with it. In this regard the diet, medicine, life circumstances, and spiritual practices that may be dharmic for one person may not be right for another. This principle of svadharma underlies Ayurveda's emphasis upon constitutional types and individualized lifestyle regimens and yoga's idea of an individualized or personalized practice. On this dharmic foundation, let us examine the spiritual, philosophical and cosmological background behind these two great systems.

Brahman/Supreme Reality

All dharmas are ultimately one in the Supreme Dharma, which is the unity of all existence. There is one Absolute Truth behind the universe, an eternal, infinite and immutable Reality called *Brahman*. Brahman means the Vast, or that which carries everything, and is the basis of all dharmic principles. Brahman is the underlying substance of existence, both manifest and unmanifest, which is not material but spiritual. We all arise from Brahman, abide in it, and must eventually return to it. All the endless and innumerable universes are nothing but waves on the sea of this infinite Being.

Brahman is Being-Consciousness-Bliss (*Sacchidananda*). Being must be conscious because an unconscious being would be a mere thing, a circumscribed or limited object. It could have no independent existence and hence no real being. Consciousness must be happy or it would not want to exist. A miserable state of consciousness would naturally put an end to itself in the course of time. Therefore, these three factors are really one.

We know Brahman or Absolute Truth only by becoming one with it, which means becoming one with the sacred ground of Being beyond the variations of name and form in the external world. We all possess an intuitive sense of this supreme reality and naturally seek it once we withdraw from egoistic involvement. Many great sages and yogis have realized it and become immortal.

Atman, The Universal Self

As Brahman pervades all things, it also exists within us as our own true being. As the original state of creatures it is our own original nature. Pure existence is also pure consciousness. This is the *Atman*, or higher Self, that dwells in the hearts of all beings. Brahman and Atman, the Absolute and the Self, are not two. They are two ways of looking at the same reality that is both in the entire universe and in each individual. The infinite Brahman knows itself as "I-am-that-I-am." To truly know oneself is to know the absolute truth, to know Brahman. But the real Self is not a personal or mental formation, not a creature or entity of any type. It is the being of consciousness that transcends time, place and individual.

To access our true Self is simple but not easy. It requires that we are at peace within our hearts and receptive to its inner light. This is the basis of meditation. Having a healthy, pure, and energetic body, prana and mind are important tools in this quest. Yoga shows us how to realize the Self. Ayurveda shows us how to live in such a way that our physical and mental actions do not deviate from it.

Samkhya, the Cosmic Science

Yoga and Ayurveda arose relative to a specific philosophical and cosmological background. Both classical yoga, the eightfold path (*Ashtanga Yoga*) taught by Patanjali in the *Yoga Sutras,* and classical Ayurveda taught by Charaka and Sushruta are based upon the Samkhya school of Vedic philosophy originally taught by the sage Kapila, a figure of great antiquity. Samkhya itself projects the prime insights of Vedic and Upanishadic thought and is found to some degree in all Vedic and Vedantic systems, particularly in their cosmologies.

Samkhya is the original spiritual science behind yoga and Ayurveda. Yoga is the technology designed to realize the great truths of Samkhya and is often spoken of as a single system called "Samkhya-Yoga." Classical yoga employs Samkhya cosmology and terminology and was generally studied along with Samkhya.[2] Ayurveda bases itself on Samkhya cosmology for its world view as it uses yogic practices among its treatment methods. Samkhya postulates twenty-four primary cosmic principles (*tattvas*) to explain all processes in the universe, with the twenty-fifth as the pure consciousness beyond all manifestation.

Purusha/Pure Consciousness

Consciousness is the ultimate principle behind the universe, which in its marvelous order reflects the workings of a supreme intelligence. Pure consciousness is the source of all subjectivity or sense of self through which we feel alive and can act independently. We all feel ourselves as conscious individuals and not as mere objects or instruments. This is our connection with the *Purusha* within us, also called the Atman or higher Self.

The outer world exists to provide experience for the Purusha. The world, in the same way as objects (like a pot), is an observable phenomenon that cannot exist for its own sake but only for that of its perceiver. The world is based on intelligence; it works through the mind and follows a pattern of organic law reflecting this Pure Consciousness behind it.

However, this higher Self is distinct from the ego, or the "I am the body" idea, which in Samkhya is called *ahamkara* or the I-process. The Purusha is not an embodied self but the pure Self-nature beyond all objectivity. It is not part of creation and is not composed of any form of matter — gross, subtle or causal. It is neither body nor mind, which are interrelated parts of matter, but the underlying consciousness through which they operate, which is not limited by them. The Purusha is the substratum or conscious ground of all manifestation which shines by his reflected light. Its light, mirrored through the mind, allows perception to occur.

While the Purusha is figuratively called "he", we must remember that it contains its own *Shakti* or power of vision as its feminine aspect. As a conscious subject we cannot call the Purusha "it", although it is not limited by gender or any other external distinctions as it is beyond all form. The goal of yoga is the same as Samkhya, to return to the consciousness of the Purusha. The goal of Ayurveda is to connect our bodies and minds with the Purusha that is the true source of happiness and well-being. The ultimate healing power and the original prana come from the Purusha.[3]

God — the Cosmic Lord, Ishvara

God, the Cosmic Lord and Creator, is called *Ishvara* in Sanskrit. Ishvara is the power that creates, sustains and destroys the world through the three forms of Brahma, Vishnu and Shiva and their feminine powers of Sarasvati, Lakshmi and Kali. Ishvara works to guide the worlds, oversees the workings of the law of karma, and aids all souls in their evolution from ignorance to enlightenment.

While Ishvara is a concept similar to God in Western, culture it should be noted that Ishvara works through various gods and goddesses as the One Creator has many diverse and specific forms. Ishvara has many different names, functions and lines of approach. Ishvara can be worshipped in the feminine sense, *Ishvari*, the Divine Mother, which is the preferable form in many yogic paths, particularly those of a tantric nature.

Ishvara is not listed separately among these twenty-four principles of classical Samkhya. However, the yoga system which

Ayurveda accepts introduces Ishvara as an additional cosmic principle, a special Purusha possessed of perfect intelligence.[4] Ishvara is the original teacher or *guru* for all souls and the source of the spiritual teachings of the *Vedas*.[5] Ayurveda recognizes God as the creator and guide, whom we should all look to for healing and guidance. Seeking divine grace is an integral part of Ayurvedic practice and the Ayurvedic doctor should strive to further the divine will and work in service to it.

The Twenty-Four Cosmic Principles (Tattvas)

These twenty-four principles (tattvas) are responsible for the structure of the universe on all levels. They are the basis for the three bodies, the five *koshas* and seven chakras of our individual existence that we will discuss later in the book.

1. Prakriti/Primordial Nature

There is one ultimate substance behind whatever can be perceived in the universe of matter and mind, which is responsible for all the qualities and energies that we observe. This prime material or world mother is called *Prakriti* and is the basic substratum of the universe, both gross and subtle. Prakriti is the original form of matter or objectivity, the unmanifest essence or undifferentiated potential of all that can appear in name, form and action. Prakriti is not matter in the gross sense as solid objectivity but as the capacity for experience by the mind. It is material in the sense of being an instrument for the conscious being or Purusha. Prakriti (Primal Matter) is insentient (that is, not conscious in itself), devoid of subjectivity, a mere latent objectivity that requires the conscious power or shakti of the Purusha to animate it.

As more subtle than the mind, which is its product, the existence of Prakriti, which is of an ideal nature, can only be inferred. We should note, however, that Prakriti is different than Brahman, which is the substance not only of the world of manifestation like Prakriti, but also of Pure Consciousness, the Purusha. Brahman is the being behind both Purusha and Prakriti, which are the powers of consciousness and unconsciousness inherent within it. For this reason, Brahman is sometimes spoken of as *Para Prakriti* or the Supreme Nature, the immutable nature beyond our changing manifestation.

Prakriti means "the first power of action" and its qualities direct the entire cosmic movement. It provides the raw material out of which the different worlds and our bodies are built. It carries the karmas and *samskaras* (tendencies) through which living creatures come into existence and forms the substratum of their minds. Prakriti therefore is also called the "Unmanifest" or *Avyakta*. It contains all that can be manifest in a dormant form. On the level of Prakriti, one can perceive all beings and all worlds as pure potentials.

Like the mother of the world, which is born from its substance, Prakriti is often spoken of in the feminine tense. Prakriti and her manifestation exist to provide experience for the Purusha so that he can gain mastery over himself and come to an understanding of his true nature. She is like a mother who selflessly provides for her child and gives him challenges to help him grow. Ayurveda recognizes Prakriti as the basis of our embodiment and experience on all levels. Each one of us has an individual physical Prakriti or nature that consists of our bodily condition, and a mental Prakriti which is the condition of our mind and heart.

Prakriti is composed of the three prime qualities of *sattva*, *rajas* and *tamas*, the qualities of light, energy and matter, through which it contains intelligence, life and the power to produce material forms. These three qualities of Prakriti are the background of all the other tattvas. They are of great importance in all yogic and ayurvedic thought and will be examined specifically in the next chapter.

2. Mahat/Cosmic Intelligence

All manifestation occurs through an underlying organic cosmic intelligence. At the beginning of creation, cosmic mind comes into being in order to create the world. It contains within itself all the laws and principles, the dharmas that the manifestation must follow. The universe first arises as a meditation of cosmic intelligence and only later takes on form externally. Mahat, or Cosmic Intelligence, therefore, is the manifest form of Prakriti or Prakriti in action. It is Prakriti molded by the will of God.

Mahat literally means "the great" and refers to the great truth principles behind life. The realm of Mahat is that of the ideal creation that transcends time, the nominal as opposed to the phenomenal realm. Mahat is the Divine Mind. Through Mahat, space, time, the divine Word and the seeds of differentiation arise. It is the womb of all creation. Yet even Mahat, cosmic intelligence, is not conscious in itself, but works through the reflected light of the Purusha or pure consciousness.

In the individual soul, Mahat becomes *Buddhi*, the power of intelligence through which we can discern truth from falsehood, right from wrong, and the eternal from the transient. Buddhi is the key faculty of our nature through which we can discover the real nature of things as apart from their changing appearances. It is the intelligence of the individual soul. Buddhi is the part of the mind that can become enlightened and reveal the higher Self, once it is redirected from outer attachments.

Attunement of individual intelligence (buddhi) with cosmic intelligence (Mahat) is the main Vedic way of knowing and the basis of Vedic insight. Yoga emphasizes the cultivation of the buddhi, Buddhi-Yoga, for developing equanimity and balance of mind for Self-realization. Ayurveda stresses cultivating a proper buddhi or intelligence so that we can learn how the mind and the body function in order to use them correctly. In the ayurvedic view, the main cause of disease is wrong functioning of the buddhi owing to the influence of the ego, which results in bad judgment, wrong values and false beliefs. Mahat and buddhi are the intelligent portion of the mind. Using the term "mind" in this sense, mind or intelligence is the origin of all the universe.

3. Ahamkara/Ego

All manifestation is a process of division through which separate creatures and different objects come into being. To enable multiplicity to occur, cosmic creation works through various separate entities or individual identities which are the basis for the ego.

Ahamkara means literally the "I-fabrication", as the ego is a process, not an intrinsic reality. It is a series of divisive thoughts but not a real entity in itself. It is a necessary power of division inherent in nature, a stage in evolution, but does not represent the underlying truth or nature of creatures. It allows the soul to identify with different bodies, but does not reveal our true Self, which is awareness beyond all embodiment.

Through ego, the basic energies latent in matter (Prakriti) and the fundamental laws contained in cosmic intelligence (Mahat) take specific forms. Under the pointed focus of the ego, the basic qualities of Nature diversify into the three groups of five: five senses, five organs of action, and five elements. These arise from ahamkara through the three *gunas* of sattva, rajas and tamas. Ego creates the mind and senses, which are the instruments that allow the individual to function. Hence ego represents the outgoing aspect of the mind, while buddhi or intelligence is its internal aspect. However, buddhi remains under the dominance of the ego unless we learn how to meditate.

Under the influence of ego, the possibility of divergence from nature arises. Prakriti or the natural condition of things can become *vikriti* — the diseased, disturbed, unnatural or artificial condition. The blindness and attachment caused by the ego is the main cause of spiritual, mental and physical disorders (except those born naturally of time). Ayurveda places much emphasis on understanding the ego and its inherent biases so that our judgment remains balanced and our actions are for the universal good, which is ultimately our own good as well. Dissolving the ego cures all psychological diseases and many physical diseases as well.

4. Manas/Outer Mind

The world manifestation works through various individual mentalities or externally directed minds. Ego automatically projects a sensory mind as it looks outward. The mind then gives rise to the five sense organs and five motor organs. The outer mind is itself the sixth sense organ and sixth motor organ and works to coordinate both. There must be an underlying power of attention to allow for the coordination of the sense and motor organs. This is the role of *manas,* which is the central circuit board for the senses. Manas means the formulating principle (from the root "man", to form) and is the principle of emotion, sensation and imagination.

Manas arises from the general sattvic and rajasic qualities of ahamkara. It possesses sattva (the power of illumination), which works through the sense organs, but also rajas (the capacity for action), which works through the motor organs. This allows manas to coordinate both sense and motor organs which arise from the specific sattvic and rajasic qualities of ahamkara as reflected through the five elements.

Prakriti, Buddhi, Ahamkara and Manas

These four principles make up the subjective aspect of creation. We have an underlying mental nature, an intelligence, an ego and a sense mind. These four work together. Unless we learn the art of meditation we may not be able to discriminate between them.

According to Samkhya, the mind itself is something material. It is observable as an object and not the true source of consciousness. Our sensory perceptions are easy to see as objects, but we can also observe our emotions and thoughts, which means that these are similarly outside our true Self. Even the ego can be observed, as when we look at our pride or fear, which shows that it also is an object and not our true Self, which is pure awareness only. Yoga shows us how to move from the mind and all of its involvement to this ever free inner Self.[6]

5 - 9. The Five Tanmatras — Sensory Potentials or Subtle Elements

The three gunas are the causal energies of creation behind the mind and consist of qualities or ideas only — balance (sattva), motion (rajas), and resistance (tamas). On a subtle level they give rise to a new set of substances, forms or impressions. These are the root energies of sound, touch, sight, taste and smell. They are called *tanmatras*, "primal measures", and are named after their corresponding sensory qualities.

1) *Shabda Tanmatra* — tanmatra of sound — ether

2) *Sparsha Tanmatra* — tanmatra of touch — air

3) *Rupa Tanmatra* — tanmatra of sight — fire

4) *Rasa Tanmatra* — tanmatra of taste — water

5) *Gandha Tanmata* — tanmatra of smell — earth

Yet the tanmatras are more subtle than our ordinary physical sensations, which derive from them. They can be experienced directly in the mind as the five main ways of knowing reality. They are emitted on a subtle level by all things in the world. They are the subtle forms of the five elements before their differentiation into gross objects. For this reason, they are sometimes called the "subtle elements." The tanmatras are connected to prana, the vital force, which is the subtle energy behind the elements. In this regard the tanmatras are connected to the doshas of Ayurveda, which reflect not only the gross elements but also the subtle elements.

The tanmatras show the basic fivefold structure of the cosmos. There cannot be a sixth sense organ or sixth element because there is no tanmatra to allow for its manifestation. Such prime energies are necessary to allow for the coordination of the sense organs with the sense objects. We can perceive various sense objects with our sense organs because both the organs and their objects are products of tanmatras, which they give off.

While the tanmatras create the manifest worlds in their seed form, in which they merge back into the gunas, they make up the causal or ideal world, the world of ideas prior to any embodiment.

10 - 14. The Five Sense Organs (Pancha Jnanendriyani)

The senses organs represent the five potentials for experience of the outer world that are latent in all minds. They are not only individual but cosmic and merely become localized in the sense organs of various creations. The sense organs pervade the cosmic ether and become manifest in individual beings. They become differentiated and developed through the process of cosmic evolution. Each corresponds to a particular sense quality (tanmatra) and element.

1) ear — organ of sound — ether

2) skin — organ of touch — air

3) eye — organ of sight — fire

4) tongue — organ of taste — water

5) nose — organ of smell — earth

The sense organs, also called organs of knowledge, are receptive only, not expressive. Their activity occurs through the corresponding organs of action. The sense organs are the vehicles through which we take in tanmatras that feed us on a subtle level. Subtle or inner forms of these organs also exist beyond the limitations of the physical body and their action gives extrasensory perception (ESP).

15 - 19. The Five Motor Organs (Pancha Karmendriyani)

Five organs of action correspond to the five sense organs and five elements.

1) mouth (expression) — ether — sound

2) hand (grasping) — air — touch

3) feet (motion) — fire — sight

4) urino-genital (emission) — water — taste

5) anus (elimination) — earth — smell

The five organs of action or motor organs allow various actions to occur. The physical organs are just structures to enable them to function in the physical world. The body is a vehicle designed to allow for certain actions to be accomplished, to allow for the mind to gain experience. These potentials for action are also found everywhere in nature and manifest in many different ways. Our physical differentiation of them is only one way. Subtle or inner forms of these organs also exist, allowing for direct action with the mind and psychic powers like telekinesis (action by thought or at a distance).

The motor organs are expressive only, not receptive. Their

capacity for reception is through the sense organs. The motor organs are more connected with the five gross elements upon which they work, while the sense organs correspond more to the tanmatras or subtle elements. The motor organs reflect the activity of prana or the life-force.

20 - 24. The Five Elements (Pancha Mahabhutani)

The five great elements are earth, water, fire, air and ether. They represent the solid, liquid, radiant, gaseous and etheric forms of matter which make up the outer world of experience, including the physical body. The sense organs and organs of action work upon them in receptive and active roles respectively.

Yet the elements as principles of density apply to all mediums and have their actions relative to the mind and vital force as well. Earth, on one hand, is a completely dense medium that allows for no evident movement. Ether, on the other hand, is a completely subtle or receptive medium that allows complete freedom of movement. Between these two polarities are all possible densities, affording the complete range of experience and the manifestation of all ideas. The five elements themselves are also manifestations of ideas. They are different densities or fields of expression for different ideas:

1) EARTH manifests the idea of solidity or stability, giving resistance in action.

2) WATER manifests the idea of liquidity or flowing motion, allowing for life.

3) FIRE manifests the idea of light, allowing for perception and for movement from place to place.

4) AIR manifests the idea of subtle movement, manifesting ideas of direction, velocity and change and giving the basis for thought.

5) ETHER manifests the idea of connection, allowing for interchange between all material mediums, communication and self expression.

To put it another way, ether manifests the idea of space, air that of time, fire that of light, water that of life, and earth that of form. Like the different lines and colors of an artist, these are the different mediums necessary for Cosmic Intelligence to express itself.

The five elements may mean not only their gross forms but their subtle and causal forms as well, their sensory counterparts and underlying ideas, making the elements encompass all forces of manifestation of soul, mind and body. In this way, the five elements are a model for all substances in the universe. Sometimes Prakriti is considered to be composed of the five elements, with the Purusha or Atman as the sixth element, the element of pure consciousness.

The twenty-four principles are not only maps of the universe, they are maps of the psyche. We will make this clearer when we discuss the three bodies and the five sheaths.

THE COSMIC PRINCIPLES: TATTVAS

Purusha	Ishvara - Cosmic Lord	Prakriti - 3 Gunas
Causal Body	Mahat, Buddhi - Individual Soul	Ego, Ahamkara
Subtle Body	Outer Mind, Manas	5 Subtle Motor Organs
	5 Pranas	5 Subtle Sense Organs
	5 Tanmatras Subtle Elements)	
Physical Body	Three Doshas	5 Gross Motor Organs
	5 Gross Sense Organs	5 Gross Elements

3

The Three Gunas
and Mental Nature

Sattva, Rajas and Tamas, the qualities born of Nature
bind the immortal soul in the body.

BHAGAVAD GITA XIV.5

Primal Nature and the Three Gunas

Primal Nature, Prakriti, is not an homogenous substance but the seed ground of multiplicity. She is like the tail of a peacock, which when withdrawn disappears into uniformity but when unfolded reveals all the colors of the rainbow. Prakriti holds in herself all the forms of creation which manifest through her three main qualities, the gunas of sattva, rajas and tamas.

Rajas is the active, stimulating or positive force that initiates change, disturbing the old equilibrium. Tamas is the passive, obstructing or negative force which sustains previous activity. Sattva is the neutral or balancing force, harmonizing the positive and negative, which oversees and observes. All three forces are necessary in ordinary activity but have spiritual implications as well.

Sattva is the quality of light, love and life, the higher or spiritual force that allows us to evolve in consciousness. It imparts dharmic virtues of faith, honesty, self-control, modesty and truthfulness. Rajas is the quality of twilight, passion, and agita-

27

tion, the intermediate or vital force, which lacks stability or consistency. It gives rise to emotional fluctuations of attraction and repulsion, fear and desire, love and hate. Tamas is the quality of darkness, non-feeling and death, the lower or material force, which drags us down into the ignorance and attachment. It causes dullness, inertia, heaviness, emotional clinging and stagnation.

Unmanifest Prakriti holds these three qualities in equilibrium, in which rajas and tamas are merged into sattva. In manifestation, the three qualities differentiate, with sattva giving rise to the mind, rajas generating the life-force, and tamas creating form and substance through which the physical body comes into being.

Laws of the Gunas

There are two basic laws of the gunas that are crucial in understanding their workings. The first law of the gunas is "the law of alternation." The three gunas are ever in dynamic interaction. All three forces remain intertwined, affecting each other in various ways. Rajas and tamas exist in the field of sattva, tamas and sattva are found in the field of rajas, and sattva and rajas move in the field of tamas. The essence of the three qualities is their interplay. We rarely see pure tamas, pure rajas or pure sattva. We must ever be ready for the gunas to change.

The second law of the gunas is "the law of continuity." The gunas tend to hold their particular natures for a certain period once they come into dominance. Substances stabilize on the level of one of the three gunas. While it is initially is difficult for tamas to become rajas, or for rajas to become sattva, once they do so they will continue in that same quality.

We can see these two laws in any movement of time. Night as darkness belongs to tamas, sunrise and sunset as transitional periods relate to rajas, and day as light corresponds to sattva.

These three phases must ever alternate. Night gives way to dawn, which in turn gives way to day, which in turn at dusk gives way to the night again in an ever-moving cycle. This is the law of alteration.

However, once a particular phase is created, it will endure with little change for a period of time. The night continues on for some time before changing into the day, which in turn has its period of duration. During these respective periods certain conditions persist. For example, we are active throughout the day and sleep through most of the night.

In this regard tamas and sattva have more continuity than rajas. Rajas, which is inherently unstable, cannot hold its own condition for long and must revert to tamas or advance to sattva. Rajas is transitional and governs the interaction between the gunas. Nevertheless, it is possible for people to remain at the level of rajas as the dominant quality for most of their lives. This is the condition of modern society, which is predominantly rajasic, active and changeable. But for rajas to continue there must be ongoing action and stimulation to sustain it.

As the gunas are relational conditions, we must remember that what is sattva on one level may become rajas or tamas relative to another. Anything that raises a person up in consciousness is sattva for them. What brings them down is tamas. This means that the more we advance along the spiritual path, what was previously sattvic or helpful may have to be discarded as tamasic as we move on to a new level.

Cultivation of Sattva

Yoga and Ayurveda emphasize the development of sattva. In yoga, sattva is the higher quality that allows spiritual growth to occur. In Ayurveda, sattva is the state of balance that makes healing happen.

Yoga practice has two stages: the development of sattva and the transcendence of sattva. Development of sattva means purification of body and mind. Transcendence of sattva means going beyond the body and mind to our true Self beyond manifestation. The general rule is that if one has not developed sattva, one cannot go beyond it. One should not forget this important rule. If we don't have the appropriate sattva or purity in our body and mind, including in our emotions, it may be premature for us to seek any higher enlightenment. Development of sattva occurs through right diet, physical purification, control of the senses, control of the mind, mantra and devotion. Transcendence of sattva comes from higher meditation practices.

Sattva is also the key to ayurvedic healing. Ayurveda states that the sattvic body and mind are less likely to suffer from disease and more able to continue in a state of balance. Disease, particularly of a chronic nature, is a tamasic state. Tamas brings about the accumulation of toxins and waste materials on a physical level and of negative thoughts and emotions on a psychological level. Health is a sattvic state of balance and adaptation which prevents any excess from occurring. Rajas is the movement either from health to disease or disease to health depending upon its direction of development. Acute diseases fall under rajas, which is pain.

However, we must not forget the admixtures of the gunas. There is a higher rajas and tamas in the field of sattva and a lower sattva in the fields of rajas and tamas. Similarly there are rajasic aspects of tamas and tamasic aspects of rajas. The following are some brief descriptions.

Rajasic Sattva: the active or transformative force of sattva, the power of spiritual aspiration that struggles upward, ever seeking greater growth and unfoldment. It is also any energy of healing that brings about integration and wholeness.

Tamasic Sattva: the destructive force of sattva that eliminates negativity. It is also the stability inherent in sattva, its capacity to endure through all obstacles. It is the capacity of a state of balance to sustain itself and to ward off disease or imbalance.

Sattvic Rajas: the type of religion, spirituality or idealism of rajasic people. It has rajasic traits of aggression, outer expansion and the seeking of power. Religions based upon militance, exclusivism and intolerance reflect this quality.

Tamasic Rajas: the inertia of rajasic types, their resistance to any higher force, and holding to their own personal power and impulses regardless of the consequences for themselves or others.

Sattvic Tamas: the religion, spirituality or idealism of tamasic people. It has tamasic traits of destruction, darkness, and delusion. It is the level of dark cults and superstitions.

Rajasic Tamas: the aggression and violence of dull and ignorant people. It is perhaps the most destructive gunic quality. Tamasic types literally trample over others and, devoid of sensitivity, delight in harm and destruction. Deep sexual perversions come at this level.

The Higher Rajasic Force

The higher rajasic force or rajasic sattva is perhaps the key force both in spirituality and healing. The lower rajasic force is rajas leading to tamas, like the dusk moving into night, or autumn becoming winter. The higher rajasic force is rajas leading to sattva, like the dawn creating the day, or spring moving into summer. In human behavior, the lower rajas is self-centered activity leading to exhaustion or suffering (tamas). The higher rajas is spiritual practice leading to peace (sattva).

For spiritual growth this higher force of rajas is necessary. It is the real shakti or transforming energy. Through it one becomes a spiritual warrior and can do spiritual practices with great energy and vigor. Yoga is not only about developing sattva but also about developing the higher rajasic force in order to bring about sattva. Similarly, Ayurveda may use strong healing methods, like powerful herbs or pancha karma to restore health. For either health or spiritual growth to occur, such a higher force of rajas or active energy of transformation is crucial. The higher force of rajas (sattvic rajas) generates the kundalini shakti or serpent power that awakens the subtle body. Kundalini systematically merges everything into pure sattva.

Tamasic sattva, the resistance power of sattva guna, is also helpful at times. In the spiritual life it helps us resist any efforts to draw us away from the path. In healing it sustains the immune functions of both body and mind.

Mental Constitution According to the Three Gunas

Ayurveda and yoga use the three gunas for determining individual mental or spiritual nature. Generally one guna predominates in our nature. However, we all have spiritual or sattvic moments, rajasic or disturbed periods, and tamasic or dull times which may be shorter or longer depending upon our nature. We also have sattvic, rajasic or tamasic phases of life which may last for months or even years.

The gunas show our mental and spiritual state through which we can measure our propensity for psychological problems. The following test is a good index of these qualities and how they work within our life and character. The answers on the left indicate sattva, in the middle rajas, and on the right tamas. Please fill out this form carefully and honestly. After answering the questionnaire for yourself, you should have someone who knows you well, like your husband, wife or close friend, fill it out for you also. Note the difference between how you view yourself and how others see you.

For most of us, our answers will generally fall in the middle or rajasic area, which is the main spiritual state in our active and outgoing culture today. We will have various psychological problems but can usually deal with them. A sattvic nature shows a spiritual disposition with few psychological issues. A highly sattvic nature is rare at any time and shows a saint or a sage. A tamasic person has a danger of severe psychological problems but would be unlikely to fill out such a chart or even read such a book. The areas in ourselves that we can improve from tamas to rajas or from rajas to sattva will aid in our peace of mind and spiritual growth. We should do all we can to make such changes.

MENTAL CONSTITUTION CHART

Diet	Vegetarian	Some Meat	Heavy Meat Diet
Drugs, Alcohol & Stimulants	Never	Occasionally	Frequently
Sensory Impressions	Calm, Pure	Mixed	Disturbed
Need for Sleep	Little	Moderate	High
Sexual Activity	Low	Moderate	High
Conrol of Senses	Good	Moderate	Weak
Speech	Calm and Peaceful	Agitated	Dull
Cleanliness	High	Moderate	Low
Work	Selfless	For Personal Goals	Lazy

MENTAL CONSTITUTION CHART (cont'd)

Anger	Rarely	Sometimes	Frequently
Fear	Rarely	Sometimes	Frequently
Desire	Little	Some	Much
Pride	Modest	Some Ego	Vain
Depression	Never	Sometimes	Frequently
Love	Universal	Personal	Lacking in Love
Violent Behavior	Never	Sometimes	Frequently
Attachment to Money	Little	Some	A lot
Contentment	Usually	Partly	Never
Forgiveness	Forgives Easily	With effort	Holds long term grudges
Concentration	Good	Moderate	Poor
Memory	Good	Moderate	Poor
Will Power	Strong	Variable	Weak
Truthfullness	Always	Most of the Time	Rarely
Honesty	Always	Most of the Time	Rarely
Peace of Mind	Generally	Partly	Rarely
Creativity	High	Moderate	Low

MENTAL CONSTITUTION CHART (cont'd)

Spiritual Study	Daily	Occasionally	Never
Mantra, Prayer	Daily	Occasionally	Never
Meditation	Daily	Occasionally	Never
Service	Much	Some	None
TOTAL	Sattva_____	Rajas_____	Tamas_____

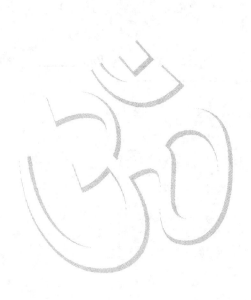

4

The Dance of the Doshas

Ayurvedic Constitution and Yoga

Vata, Pitta and Kapha are called the three supports.
Knowing this group of three as the sacred threefold
mantra OM, the wise are liberated.

BRIHAT YOGI YAJNAVALKYA SMRITI II.25

The Three Great Cosmic Forces

The entire universe derives from three original powers of energy, light and matter. Science recognizes these as physical forces governing the external world but, from a Vedic standpoint, they are powers of consciousness itself. Energy is the origin of the life force that is the most powerful of all forces. Light is the origin of the mind, through which we can see, know and discern. Matter is the basis of the body through which we have a form and substance in time and space.

These three powers work through the three central elements. Energy and life work through the element of air, which is active in nature, stimulating all things to motion. Air or wind is not simply an atmospheric force, but exists throughout nature as various currents and attractions arising through space. Space is not empty but is teeming with active energies at an invisible level. There is a solar wind,[7] for example, and interstellar gases and their flows. The nerve force in the body is a kind of wind and the mind's force also travels like a breath of air.

Light and intelligence function through the element of fire, which gives illumination. There are many forms of light — from the galaxies, stars and planets in the external world to the lights of the senses and seeing power of the mind. Matter, particularly at a biological level, is dominated by the element of water, which provides stability and sustains the bodily tissues. Embodied life arises in water and is nourished by it. Yet on all levels a watery or cohesive force serves to hold things together.

These three forces, when imbued with prana or the life-force, create the three doshas: *Vata*, *Pitta* and *Kapha*, the air, fire and water humors. Vata, as wind, imparts energy, life, movement and expression. Pitta, as fire, creates heat and light, through which we have vision, digestion, and transformation. Kapha, as water, contains, supports and nourishes the other two forces as living tissue.

Energy ultimately is the force of God, the Divine Will that rules all actions in the universe. It is not merely a blind or inanimate force but the very power of consciousness. Light is Divine Intelligence that becomes the basis for the individual soul or conscious Self in creatures. This life and mind is embodied in the world through the medium of water, the worlds or realms of experience in which the soul takes birth. Energy is the spirit, which is formless. Light is the soul, which has a form dependent upon a fuel, the water that makes up the body.

An early text on yoga relates this fact.[8] Air is God, spirit or pure consciousness, the formless force and presence that pervades everything. Fire is the embodied soul, hidden in the body like fire latent in wood. The spiritual life consists of awakening the light of fire, the soul's intelligence in our heart, and lifting it out of the limited bodily sphere into the unlimited realm of the Spirit, merging our individual fire into the cosmic air and space.

The Three Doshas

Our biological existence is a dance of the three doshas of vata, pitta and kapha. Life is a multicolored tapestry of their movement in various plays of balance and imbalance, coming together and going apart. These three powers color and determine our conditions of growth and aging, health and disease. *Dosha* means a fault or a blemish and indicates the factors that bring about disease and decay.

The doshas impact us on two primary levels. First, they are the factors that produce the physical body and are responsible for its substance and its function. Our tissues are mainly kapha or watery in nature. The digestive system is mainly pitta or fire. The nervous system is mainly vata or wind. Second, one of the three doshas predominates in each individual and becomes the basic determinate of his or her particular constitution or mind-body type. In this regard, Ayurveda speaks of people as vata types, pitta types or kapha types relative to individual habits and proclivities from bodily structure to emotional responses.

In the practice of yoga, both levels of the doshas are important. First, an understanding of the doshas allows us to gauge the effects of yoga practice on both the gross and subtle bodies. Yogic views of anatomy, physiology and psychology were originally formulated in terms of the doshas. The doshas tell us how the various organs and systems of the body work from the yogic perspective of prana. They provide keys to the nadis and chakras of the subtle body. Similarly the doshas help us understand how the mind functions, as well as its connection to the soul, which follows the same energies as the body but at a deeper level.

Second, an understanding of ayurvedic constitutional types helps us adapt yoga practices according to individual requirements. The asanas, pranayama and meditation practices appropriate for one doshic type may not be useful for another.

Ayurveda enables us to personalize yoga practices to the unique energetics of different mind-body types. It not only ensures that yoga practice benefits our health but that it is able to actualize our entire human potential. Yoga practitioners should know their ayurvedic constitution for the right application of practices. Yoga teachers should have knowledge of Ayurveda to vary the practices they recommend relative to individual needs.

Ayurveda treatment occurs on two similar levels relative to the doshas. The first is treatment of disease, helping us deal with specific health complaints from common ailments to life-threatening illnesses. On this level, Ayurveda is concerned with specific therapies to reduce doshic excesses. These therapies, like the prescription of powerful herbs, are usually performed by an Ayurvedic doctor. The second level is lifestyle management. Ayurveda shows us how to live in harmony with our constitution, not only to prevent disease but also to utilize our full soul potential. On this level, Ayurveda deals with general lifestyle practices to apply in our daily lives, which rests more in our own power.

Yoga has a place in both levels of ayurvedic treatment. Yoga is a therapeutic tool of Ayurveda for both disease treatment and for lifestyle management. Yoga postures and pranayama treat a variety of ailments, particularly structural problems or low energy conditions. Yoga is also excellent for psychological and mental disorders because of its specific action on the mind through meditation. However, yoga is probably more important for lifestyle management than for treatment of disease. Yoga postures, pranayama and meditation are among the best tools for keeping our doshas in balance.

Ayurvedic books go into great detail about the functioning of the doshas and can be consulted for more information in this regard. Here we will look into the doshas relative to the practice of yoga.

Vata Dosha

Vata, which literally means wind, is the primary dosha or biological force. It is the motivating power behind the other two doshas, which are lame or incapable of movement without it. Vata is primarily ether in substance and air in motion. It exists as the air that we hold in the empty spaces of the body, like in the hollow organs, joints, and bone cavities, particularly the hips and lower back. On an inner level, vata is both the life-force and the energy of thought that moves in the space of the mind.

Vata's sense organs are the ears and skin and its motor organs are speech and the hands, which relate to the ether and air elements and tanmatras. On an inner level, vata governs sensory, emotional and mental harmony balance, and promotes mental adaptability and comprehension. Vata endows us with positive traits of creativity, enthusiasm, speed, agility and responsiveness that allow us to achieve our goals in life.

Vata's primary physical site is in the colon. Vata is a positive factor in the energy produced through the digestion of food. As a toxin or disease-causing factor, it is the excess gas resulting from faulty digestion. Disturbed vata causes mental, nervous and digestive disorders, including low energy and weakening of all bodily tissues.

Yet vata is not separate from the other doshas. Like the wind that moves with the clouds in the sky, vata contains within itself subtle particles of water and the potential of fire in the form of electric force. After all, it is changes in temperature (fire) and pressure (water) that make the wind blow. The clouds of vata generate the lightning or fire that gives rise to pitta and the watery particles or rain that give rise to kapha. Vata is the origin of the other two doshas. Proper balance of vata depends upon the right amount of pitta and kapha held within it, just as the amount of heat and water in the wind determines how it blows. The key to managing all the doshas is to care for vata. The cosmic vata, or *Vayu*, energizes and upholds dharma or cosmic law. Similarly, the proper control of vata brings dharma or natural order to all the workings of the body and mind.

Pitta Dosha

Pitta means "the power of digestion or cooking" — that which causes things to ripen and mature. As fire cannot exist directly in the body, pitta exists in the body in the medium of oily and acidic secretions and so is said to contain an aspect of water as well. Pitta is responsible for all forms of digestion and transformation in the body, from the cellular level to the workings of the gastrointestinal tract. Pitta governs digestion on mental and spiritual levels as well — our capacity to digest impressions, emotions and ideas in order to arrive at a perception of truth. Pitta endows us with positive traits of intelligence, courage and vitality. Without it we lack the decisiveness or motivation to accomplish our goals.

Pitta is located in the small intestine and stomach among the organs, the sweat and sebaceous glands, and the blood and lymph among the tissues. Its sense organ is the eyes and its motor organ is the feet, which relate to the element and tanmatra of fire. Its site of accumulation is in the small intestine, where it builds up as acidity. Pitta is produced as the positive energy or heat of the blood. As a disease factor, it manifests through excess or toxic blood that gives rises to inflammation and infection.

Pitta depends upon vata for its enervation and movement and on kapha for its support, just as fire requires both oxygen (air) and fuel in order to burn properly. It holds some degree of vata or nervous energy within it and grounds itself with the appropriate kapha or water.

Kapha Dosha

Kapha, which also indicates mucus or phlegm, means "what makes things stick together" and refers to the power of cohesion. Kapha serves as the bodily container for pitta and vata, or energy and heat. Kapha itself, as water, is held in the medium of earth, the skin and mucous linings, affording it a secondary earth element as well.

Kapha is located in the chest, throat and head in the upper body, the sites of mucus production, but also in the pancreas, sides and stomach in the middle body where fat accumulates, and in lymph and fat tissues generally. Its sense organs are taste and smell, the nose and tongue and its motor organs are the urino-genital and excretory organs which relate to the water and earth elements and tanmatras. Kapha endows us with emotion and feeling. This gives love and caring, devotion and faith, which serve to keep us in harmony internally and unite us with others. Kapha allows us to retain what we have achieved through our efforts.

Kapha's primary physical site is the stomach, where mucus is produced, which then overflows into the lungs and lymphatic system. Kapha is produced through the plasma, which is the main kapha tissue in the body, providing hydration and nourishment to all the tissues. As a disease factor, Kapha manifests through excess plasma that becomes mucus. This causes overweight, edema, lung diseases, swollen glands and other kapha disorders.

Kapha depends upon vata for its stimulation and movement. It requires pitta for its warmth. The body, though primarily composed of water (kapha), is a special form of water in which heat (pitta) and vital energy (vata) are contained. Water that is cold or does not move cannot sustain life.

The Doshas as Constitutional Factors

The Doshas create three different primary types of individual constitutions or mind-body types. No type is necessarily better or worse than the others. Each has its benefits as well as its weaknesses. Kapha types possess the strongest build but can lack in motivation and adaptation to use it properly. Vata types have the weakest build but the greatest capacity for change and adaptation to protect it. Pitta types have moderate physical strength but greater mental and emotional force.

Below is included a simple test to determine the doshas in your own nature. No person is of one type only, so expect some combination of traits. The predominant trait will determine your type.

AYURVEDIC CONSTITUTION CHART

	VATA (AIR)	PITTA (FIRE)	KAPHA (WATER)
Height:	tall or very short	medium	usually short but can be tall and large
Frame:	thin, bony good muscles	moderate, developed	large, well formed
Weight:	low, hard to hold weight	moderate	heavy, hard to lose weight
Skin Luster:	dull or dusky	ruddy, lustrous	white or pale
Skin Texture:	dry, rough, thin	warm, oily	cold, damp, thick
Eyes:	small, nervous	piercing, easily inflamed	large, white
Hair:	dry, thin	thin, oily	thick, oily, wavy, lustrous
Teeth:	crooked, poorly formed	moderate, bleeding gums	large, well formed
Nails:	rough, brittle	soft, pink	soft, white

AYURVEDIC CONSTITUTION CHART (cont'd)

	VATA (AIR)	PITTA (FIRE)	KAPHA (WATER)
Joints:	stiff, crack easily	loose	firm, large
Circulation:	poor, variable	good	moderate
Appetite:	variable, nervous	high, excessive	moderate but constant
Thirst:	low, scanty	high	moderate
Sweating:	scanty	profuse but not enduring	low to start but profuse
Stool:	hard or dry	soft, loose	normal
Urination:	scanty	profuse, yellow	moderate, clear
Sensitivites:	cold, dryness, wind	heat, sunlight, fire	cold, damp
Immune Function:	low, variable	moderate, sensitive to heat	high
Disease Tendency:	pain, inflammation	fever, edema	congestion
Disease Type	nervous	blood, liver	mucous, lungs
Activity:	high, restless	moderate	low, moves slowly
Endurance:	poor, easily exhausted	moderate but focused	high
Sleep:	poor, disturbed	variable	excess
Dreams:	frequent, colorful	moderate, romantic	infrequent, disturbed
Memory:	quick but absent-minded	sharp, clear	slow but steady
Speech:	fast, frequent	sharp, cutting	slow, melodious
Temperament:	nervous, changeable	motivated	content, conservative
Positive Emotions:	adaptability	courage	love
Negative Emotions:	fear	anger	attachment
Faith:	variable, erratic	strong, determined	steady, slow to change
TOTAL	Vata____	Pitta____	Kapha____

Biological and Spiritual Nature

The Three Gunas and the Three Doshas

Yoga examines individuals in terms of their mental/spiritual level according to the three gunas. Ayurveda looks at individuals in terms of their psychophysical constitution through the three doshas. Yet Ayurveda also considers the role of the gunas as factors of mental health and well-being and yoga considers the doshas relative to physiological functioning. For a complete ascertainment of the individual nature, both the gunic and doshic natures must be considered.

The doshas are a biological classification that is horizontal in application, with no necessary spiritual implications. A vata type may be a saint or a sinner; the same is the case with the other two types. The gunas are a spiritual classification that is vertical in nature. It has no necessary physical implications. A saint or sinner may be vata, pitta or kapha in body.

Putting these two classifications together like horizontal and vertical lines, we can arrive at a precise indication of where a person is at in life. Please do both the dosha and guna tests to see how these two factors combine in your nature, not only to learn if you are vata, pitta or kapha, but also to see if the dosha is at a level of sattva, rajas or tamas. The following types show such typical indications.

Vata Spiritual Types

Sattvic Vata types are creative and open-minded, with broad comprehension of diverse topics and quick understanding of many points of view. They are excellent communicators with mobile and enthusiastic minds and personalities. They possess a strong sense of human unity, are receptive and sensitive to others. They have a strong healing energy, abundant vitality, and are a source of constant inspiration.

Rajasic Vata types are ever active, expressive and on the move, striving to achieve various and changing goals in life. Always restless and full of desire, they want to do more and more and can never rest satisfied with anything. They are easily distracted, pursuing novelty, and may become hyperactive and inconsistent. Coming on quickly like the wind, they can be overly talkative, superficial, noisy, and disruptive.

Tamasic Vata types exhibit a deceptive, fearful and erratic behavior that easily becomes extreme, going against any order or courtesy. They are inclined to theft, prone to sexual perversions, easily addicted to drugs and other escapes, and sometimes suicidal. They cannot be trusted with anything serious and play havoc with all whom they encounter.

Pitta Spiritual Types

Sattvic Pitta types display higher qualities of light, intelligence and warmth, shining like the sun on everyone. They are disciplined, perceptive and discriminating in their thinking, always considering the point of view of others. They are friendly and courageous in their actions, with warmth and compassion for all. They function as natural leaders with strong wills for growth and development.

Rajasic Pitta types aim at achievement and success, often regardless of the means or the method. They promote themselves and their agendas with skill and determination, not stopping until they have reached their goal of power and position. They are critical and controlling, prone to anger and intolerance. This leads them to be reckless and vain, which can bring about their downfall.

Tamasic Pitta types are destructive and violent in their emotions and behavior. They harbor much hatred, resentment and hostility in life and take it out on anyone who gets in their way. They do not respect any social laws or the feelings of others. Most criminal leaders and underworld figures are of this type. They may be paranoid or psychopathic and should be avoided at all cost.

Kapha Spiritual Types

Sattvic Kapha types exhibit kapha virtues of love, devotion, faith and contentment, which gives them a comforting presence to all who come into contact with them. They have much steadiness, patience, equanimity and balance of mind. They are loyal, forgiving, nurturing and supportive. They view all creatures with the eyes of a caring parent and provider.

Rajasic Kapha types aim at acquisition and like to dominate others through controlling material resources. They are greedy and materialistic, seeking wealth and position for themselves and their family. Their goal is to accumulate all the good things of life, from home and clothes to property and assets of all types. They are driven to own and accumulate and are not satisfied until their possessions overwhelm them.

Tamasic Kapha types are caught in inertia and stagnation, which often manifests as various addictions. Their minds are dull and insensitive and they are usually depressed. They refuse to make efforts in life and are incapable of self-reflection, preferring to blame others for their predicaments. They trample over others in their heaviness and lethargy. Their bodies similarly are usually overweight and full of toxins.

5

The Paths of Yoga

Yoga is severing the connection with that which causes suffering. Yoga should be practiced with insight and with an unperturbed heart.

BHAGAVAD GITA VI. 23

Raja Yoga, the Integral Path

The system of classical yoga was compiled by Patanjali in the *Yoga Sutras*, based upon older traditions going back to Vedic times. Called Raja Yoga or the Royal Yoga, it covers the entire range of yogic practices from asana and pranayama to mantra and the many forms of meditation. This integral yoga parallels an integral Ayurveda that similarly deals with all aspects of our nature from body to soul and all possible healing methods from food to meditation.

According to Patanjali, "Yoga is the complete control of the operations of the mind."[9] These operations of the mind, called *vrittis*, constitute all our mental activities from the deepest subconscious memories to the highest superconscious insights. Patanjali is not referring to control of the mind in the ordinary sense but to a complete mastery of all levels of consciousness, including subliminal and cosmic layers not known to ordinary awareness or even to modern psychology.

Only from such control of the mind can arise knowledge of our true Self (Atman or Purusha) beyond manifestation,[10] which is the ultimate goal of yoga practice. The silent mind becomes a mirror that reveals our real Self, whose nature is pure awareness. This is the state of liberation (*moksha*) in which we transcend time, space and karma and enter into the infinite, eternal and self-existent. Yet to reach this control of the mind we must have mastery of the body, senses and prana, as well as the outer aspects of our personal and social life. For this reason, yoga does not neglect even common factors of diet and emphasizes the relevance of Ayurveda.

The Eight Limbs of Yoga

Raja Yoga provides an integral eightfold approach or eight limbs (*ashtanga*) for the development of consciousness. These are like the limbs of the body and work together in various ways. Each has its proper role necessary for right development, though all are not of equal importance.

Eight Limbs of Yoga

1) *Yama* — Rules of Social Conduct

2) *Niyama* — Rules of Personal Behavior

3) *Asana* — Physical Postures

4) *Pranayama* — Control of the Vital Force

5) *Pratyahara* — Control of the Senses

6) *Dharana* — Right Attention or Control of the Mind

7) *Dhyana* — Meditation

8) *Samadhi* — Absorption

The first five limbs — from yama to pratyahara — make up the outer aspect of yoga. They are preliminary in nature, laying the foundation for deeper practice. The first two (yama and niyama) refer to the right attitudes, values and lifestyle practices necessary for yoga, its ethical foundation. The next three (asana, pranayama, pratyahara) are the means to control the outer aspects of our nature as body, breath and senses. The last three (dharana, dhyana and samadhi) are called *samyama* or integration. They naturally go together. Attention naturally leads to meditation, which in time results in absorption or the unification of the perceiver and the perceived. They bring us knowledge of our true Self.

Ayurveda harmonizes the body and prana to enable us to proceed with the inner process of meditation. It is mainly part of the outer aids of yoga. However, ayurvedic healing for the mind also involves the inner aspects of yoga like mantra and meditation. Ayurveda therefore shares the same scope as yoga but with a different orientation and purpose.

1 & 2. Yama and Niyama: The Dharmic Foundation of Yoga and Ayurveda

The yamas or dharmic principles of social behavior are nonviolence (*ahimsa*), truthfulness (*satya*), control of sexual energy (*brahmacharya*), non-stealing (*asteya*) and non-clinging (*anabhinivesha*). These establish right interaction with other human beings and our external environment.

Right social behavior is important for health, psychological well-being and spiritual development. If we follow these observances, we will have no harmful impact upon the world and not get entangled in external complications of wrong relationships or wrong possessions. The yamas also are a code for physicians: not to cause harm, to tell the truth, not to get sexually involved with patients, not to charge undue fees for treatment, and not to be attached to one's practice or its results.

The niyamas or dharmic principles of personal behavior are contentment (*santosha*), purity (*shaucha*), self-study (*svadhyaya*), self-discipline (*tapas*), and surrender to God (*Ishvara pranidhana*). These are the lifestyle principles necessary to establish a personal yogic practice in life. They are also the basis of ayurvedic life regimens for constitution balancing. Purity includes vegetarian diet and physical detoxification. Surrender to the divine is the key to sustaining all these practices, which cannot be achieved by mere personal effort. The last three — self-discipline, self-study, and surrender to God — are the foundation of *Kriya Yoga*, the yoga of internal action that renders one fit for samadhi.[11]

Yama and niyama constitute the dharmic or ethical foundation for all right living, including the health practices of Ayurveda. These two sets of principles go together. Unless we have integrity in our social interactions, we cannot have it in our personal behavior and vice versa.

3. Asana

Asana means right posture or posture in harmony with our inner consciousness. Its aim is a sustained and comfortable sitting posture to facilitate meditation. Asanas bring balance and harmony to the physical body, particularly the musculoskeletal system that is the support of the body. Asana is part of the ayurvedic treatment system for the physical body. Postures can be used to increase vitality or to balance the doshas. They can be adjusted to target certain organs or weak spots in the body. Asana is a subject of a separate chapter in the book.

4. Pranayama

Pranayama means not simply breath control but the controlled expansion of the life-force. It is not the suppression of the breath, which is harmful, but contacting higher sources of prana both within and around us. Pranayama consists of deepening and extending the prana until it leads to a condition of peace. When the prana is at peace, the life-force and through it the senses, emotions and mind are put to rest. Pranayama is another important ayurvedic method for increasing vigor and vitality and promoting the power of healing. The issue of prana and the practice of pranayama are dealt with in several chapters.

5. Pratyahara

Pratyahara is not simply closing off the senses but right management of the senses and the ability to go beyond them. It is not suppression of the senses but their right application, which includes the ability to put them to rest. Ayurveda regards all diseases as based upon the wrong use of the senses. How we use our senses determines the kind of energy we take in from the external world to feed our minds, which either nourishes or deranges us.

Pratyahara techniques involve either shutting off the senses, like closing the eyes or ears, or using our senses with attention rather than distraction. This includes various forms of mantra or visualization. Inner sensory sources may be tapped like the inner sounds (*nada*) that provide subtle kinds of impressions. A special chapter is also devoted to pratyahara.

6. Dharana

Dharana is control of the mind, which is right attention. It is the capacity to give all our mental energy at will to whatever we need to examine. Dharana involves developing and extending our power of our attention. Dharana techniques consists of various ways of directing or controlling our attention, like concentration on particular objects or ideas. Common dharana techniques including concentration on the five chakras and their ruling elements. A second method is to concentrate the mind in the heart. A third method is to concentrate the outer space in the inner space that dwells within the heart. Dharana is mentioned in several contexts later in the book.

7. Dhyana

Dhyana is meditation, which is our capacity to sustain our attention without distraction. Meditation enables us to mirror reality and objectively perceive the truth of things. Meditation may be on an external object, like the ocean, the sky, or a statue of a deity. It may be on an internal object that we visualize like a deity or a yantra. It may be on an idea or truth principle, like infinity or oneness. It may be without form altogether and totally open. It may be active, pursuing a line of thought or inquiry, or passive, merely observing.

Meditation in the highest sense is not a technique. Meditation techniques more properly belong to pratyahara or dharana. True meditation is the natural state of awareness, not a method. But this requires some preparation to reach, as indicated by the other limbs of yoga. A separate chapter is also devoted to meditation.

8. Samadhi

Samadhi, which we could call absorption, is the capacity to become one with the object of our perception. It is the unity of the perceiver and the perceived in direct perception, through which the nature of ultimate reality can be clearly known. Samadhi is our capacity to merge with things in consciousness that shows our joy and fulfillment in life. It brings us to the underlying Divine nature in all things. It is the natural outcome of true meditation. Samadhi or union is the goal of all that we seek. Yoga does this inwardly so that we can be one with all.

The Paths of Yoga

In yoga there is no insistence that all individuals must follow one path or another. Yoga encourages us to follow the path that most appeals to our heart. There are many different paths and styles of yoga relative to different individual inclinations and the different aspects of our nature. This is similar to Ayurveda, which teaches various diets and life regimens according to different constitutional types. These paths of yoga can be summarized under five different areas. Raja Yoga includes all the main yogic paths, but these can be pursued separately as well.

1) *Jnana Yoga* — Yoga of Knowledge

2) *Bhakti Yoga* — Yoga of Devotion

3) *Kriya Yoga*, including Hatha Yoga — Yoga of Technique

4) *Karma Yoga* — Yoga of Service

5) *Raja Yoga* — Integral Yoga, combining all four

1. The Yoga of Knowledge, Jnana Yoga

Yoga is first of all a seeking of knowledge, an inquiry into the truth of life, self, God and the universe. Yet it is a special type of inquiry, not done with the outer mind and senses but with the inner mind and heart. The yoga of knowledge is not primarily a practice of the thinking mind, though it does start out with a deep pondering of the primary questions of life and requires a rigorous rationality. It is a way of meditation that requires that the mind dwell in a state of peaceful observation to discover truth, not by thought but by perception.

The yoga of knowledge is simple in its formulation but difficult to practice. It says that God or the Absolute is our true Self. All we need to do to find God is let go of our external involvement, give up all thought, and come to rest within our hearts and we are That! Its main method is Self-inquiry (*Atma-vichara*), tracing out the origin of our thoughts to the I-thought that arises from the heart as the root of all thoughts. It also employs various other methods of reasoning, discrimination and affirmation, including special mantras like *Aham Brahmasmi*, "I am God."

Because of its directness, the yoga of knowledge is recommended mainly for the highest level of aspirant. Its foundation is complete renunciation and tremendous austerity such as few, particularly from our sensate and materialistic culture, can achieve. However, most of us can benefit from the practices of the yoga of knowledge, like silent meditation on Brahman or inquiry into the Self, even if we are not at the highest level. Yet we must support these with other yogic disciplines to insure that our development is complete. Above all, the yoga of knowledge requires complete control of the senses and pranas, which rests upon a pure diet and self-control, for which Ayurveda offers much help.

The yoga of knowledge is particularly attractive to pitta or fiery types as it rests upon a clear focus of the mind and determined insight such as they are more likely to possess. However, vata or airy types are sometimes drawn to it because of their capacity for expansive thinking and detachment from the body. Kapha or watery types occasionally follow it because their steadiness of mind allows them to develop deep peace and inner calm.

2. The Yoga of Devotion, Bhakti Yoga

Devotion is the path of divine love through which we seek to merge into the divine within the heart. It consists of the worship of the Divine Beloved as the ultimate reality, externally and internally.

Devotion takes different forms relative to how we choose to approach the divine. Yoga grants us complete freedom in choosing whatever form of God most appeals to our heart. This derives from the same recognition of individual differences and constitutional types. Yoga offers various chosen deities (*Ishta devatas*), like Shiva, Vishnu or the Goddess, or incarnations of God (*avatars*) like Rama, Krishna or Buddha. Sometimes the teacher or guru, as a symbol of the divine teacher, may become the object of worship. Deities may also reflect ayurvedic energies and be used for balancing the prana and mind. Formless devotion or devotion to divine qualities and attributes is another approach.

There are many devotional practices — the performance of rituals (*puja*), devotional songs (*kirtan*), chanting the names of God (*japa*), meditation on a form of the Divine (*upasana*), or assuming various attitudes or moods of divine worship. These are quite diverse but generally are approached spontaneously. Bhakti yoga has a certain freedom, which is the power of inspiration; therefore it is not as structured as the other yogas. However, to advance far along it requires purity, consecration and self-sacrifice to the Divine Beloved.

The yoga of devotion is the best means of healing the heart and our emotional nature, which in the modern world, with all our relationship problems, is often hurt or disturbed. This healing of the heart is emphasized in ayurvedic psychology.

Devotion appeals mainly to kapha types who are the most emotional of the three types. Kapha types have a natural love that best expresses itself through devotion. Pitta types can be devotional as well, but in their case their devotion is more determined and concentrated, like the warrior serving his king or queen. Vata types are the least devotional but benefit the most from devotion because it is the best thing for calming the heart and relieving the fear and anxiety from which they are more likely to suffer.

3. The Yoga of Service, Karma Yoga

Karma yoga refers to the yoga of work or action, which is twofold. Its first part is prayers and rituals for self-purification and the upliftment of the world. The second part is service to living beings. All spiritual teachings speak of the need to help the world and to uplift humanity. Most practitioners of yoga are expected to do some work of service, called *seva* in Sanskrit. This may consist of providing food or clothing to the poor or needy, working in schools or hospitals, or distributing books and teachings. It is not limited to helping people but extends to helping animals, plants and the planet itself, including various forms of social and political activism. Most yogic paths begin with the student taking up some karma yoga or service activity from cooking, cleaning the ashram or administration to setting up schools or hospitals.

The two aspects of karma yoga are related. All service is a divine ritual. All ritual has as its aim the upliftment of living beings. All yogas are rooted in karma yoga. One's spiritual practice should be a service to all beings or it has little value. Even liberated souls are not free from the practice of karma yoga, which compels them to return to the world to help the ignorant. Karma yoga is the beginning and the end, the lowest and the highest of all the yogas. Those who neglect it miss the real spirit of yoga.

Kapha types prefer karma yoga that takes a nurturing role, caring for others. Pitta types prefer social or political activism that projects a cause to help change the world. Vata types prefer karma yoga that engages the mind, like writing or teaching. Karma yoga is an important ayurvedic tool of psychological healing and the foundation of ayurvedic life regimens. If what we do is not a form of service, it is bound to breed physical or psychological disturbance.

4. Kriya Yoga, The Yoga of Technique

Yogic science has its own technology, consisting of various methods and techniques involving body, breath and mind, to help unfold our deeper awareness. These all fall under the yoga of technique or inner action (kriya yoga). Kriya refers to an

action, process or movement, particularly the internal unfoldment of prana and mind to bring about purification and transformation so that we are ready for deep meditation.

Kriya yoga consists of three parts: *tapas* or self-discipline,
svadhyaya or self-study, and *Ishwara-pranidhana*, surrender to
God.[12] Self-discipline creates the internal heat that helps ripen
or mature our spiritual aspiration. This includes everything from
fasting to meditation as means of developing and energizing
our will power. Self-study also means following one's own
dharma, which implies understanding one's ayurvedic constitution as well. Surrender to God is not only devotion but learning to channel the divine energy for self-improvement so that
our practice is not limited by ego constraints.

In the yogas of knowledge and devotion, techniques are
subordinated to a more primary self-observation or self-surren-
der. But most aspirants, particularly in the modern world, require a good deal of work and purification to become capable
of true insight or divine love. It is very difficult to go directly
to God or the Self even for the best people in the best of times.
To proceed without techniques can be to take the hard path,
like trying to go on foot when a good vehicle is there to speed
us on our journey. However, some people overemphasize technique, which, without knowledge or devotion, must remain
artificial and sterile. Technique should be blended with knowledge and devotion for it to best proceed and it should be done
as a form of service.

Kriya yoga appeals mainly to vata types who like movement and action. However, pitta types, who like to work with
fire and energy and have a scientific bent, may be drawn to it as
well. Kapha types are least likely to be drawn to it but benefit
greatly from more action and the movement energy that it affords. There are many aspects of the yoga of technique. Below
we list some of the main approaches.

Mantra Yoga: includes all forms of prayer, chanting and singing the praise of God. It is connected with music, poetry, symbology and mythology, which are all different levels of the mantra. All yoga paths employ some mantric approach. The yoga of knowledge uses mantras like *Aham Brahmasmi* or "I am God." The yoga of devotion employs names of God such as *Om Namo Bhagavate Vasudevaya* or "Reverence to Krishna." Karma yoga is performed while chanting devotional mantras. Yoga techniques emphasize mantras chanted along with pranayama or meditation.

Mantra is perhaps the main method of the yoga of technique. It is more important than asana and could be called asanas for the mind. All yoga and ayurvedic practice should begin and end with mantras, as well as using mantras along the way. Ayurveda considers mantra to be its most important healing method after the use of herbs, so all ayurvedic practitioners should study mantra yoga. Note special chapter on mantra.

Tantra: literally means technology and refers to various techniques or methodologies of yoga including mantra, yantra, visualization, and devotional worship, including various forms of temple worship. It is not simply sexual postures, which is merely one side of tantra and one of its lower forms. Tantra is an energetic approach teaching us how to work with energy on a subtle level. Tantra, therefore, is mainly a path of raja yoga because of its integral nature and, secondarily, a path of kriya yoga because of its practical side. Tantric yoga has been the most prevalent form of raja yoga since medieval times in India. It uses all eight limbs of Raja Yoga, adding to it specific forms and practices.

The sexual tantra is part of the *vamachara* or "left-handed" tantra that employs practices not considered to be dharmic or pure, including indulgence in sex, meat, and fish. It is considered appropriate for individuals who have not yet advanced to the stage of higher yoga practices and are still caught in desire and in the senses (*rajas* and *tamas*). As most people in the modern world are at this stage, such tantra can have great appeal and is not without its possible value. It is always important to start where we are in life. But such tantra should not be confused with higher tantric yoga practices that proceed through mantra and meditation and follow the way of renunciation.

In tantra we find the most clear description of the subtle body, its energy centers (chakras), and the higher forces like kundalini working through them. Kundalini yoga is part of tantra. Tantric methods are often combined with those of Ayurveda, particularly for purposes of healing the subtle body and rejuvenation of the physical body. Ayurvedic alchemy, the use of specially prepared mineral and mental preparations and rejuvenative herbs, is part of a tantric approach. The use of gems links not only Ayurveda and tantra but Vedic astrology (*Jyotish*) as well. Tantra combines a wealth of techniques that are quite useful for physical and psychological healing.

Hatha Yoga: is the most commonly known of the yogas of technique. It literally means the yoga of effort or force. While the tendency is to identify it with the physical yoga and asana practice, it is more than that. Classical hatha yoga texts like *Hatha Yoga Pradipika* and *Gheranda Samhita* are tantric and teach not only asana but a whole range of tantric methods of purification, mantra and meditation.

The asana-dominant yoga of the West is sometimes called hatha yoga because in hatha yoga texts we find the most detailed explanation of various asanas. In this regard, the best asana teachers and perhaps the greatest development of asana can be found in the West today. In India the main yogic path is devotion and asana is generally treated superficially.

However, Western hatha yoga seldom goes into the meditation parts of classical hatha yoga. Therefore it is not entirely correct to call it hatha yoga. Classical hatha yoga was a path for hermits, requiring great physical austerity. It employs powerful methods of internal cleansing that demand very special living circumstances. Hatha yoga is said to lead us to Raja Yoga or the higher yoga, in which meditation becomes the main concern.

Owing to its connection with the physical body, hatha yoga is closely linked with Ayurveda and describes asanas in ayurvedic terms. Ayurveda employs the asanas of hatha yoga as one of its mainly healing modalities. It also recommends various purification measures of hatha yoga for healing purposes. Hatha yoga is particularly useful for vata types who need to be more grounded in the physical body, but it is useful for the other ayurvedic types as well. However, its stronger practices should be taken up with caution as they can aggravate vata severely.

Ayurvedic Yoga

Ayurveda itself is a form of yoga. It can be called the yoga of healing. Ayurveda employs aspects of all the yogas depending upon the level, temperament and constitution of the individual to aid in their healing, right lifestyle and spiritual development. A true ayurvedic practitioner, therefore, is also be a yogi. He or she has mastery not only of the physical body but of the pranas and the mind, with knowledge of the subtle body and the soul. A true doctor heals through the life-force, not through his or her own personal energy. The mind of a true healer is attuned with the divine or the inner Self.

Ayurveda should be practiced as karma yoga, as a form of service to living beings. It should be done for the purpose of helping others, not merely for one's own personal or material benefit. Without this sense of service, the spiritual side of

Ayurveda cannot grow in a person.

An ayurvedic adept should possess a good knowledge of hatha yoga and its understanding of posture, breath and awareness. Yet Ayurveda also employs the techniques of raja yoga for healing the subtle body and soul. Those studying Ayurveda should examine the *Yoga Sutras* as well and have a knowledge of its system and application.

Ayurveda uses mantra yoga as a means not only of healing but of projecting all healing energies. Ayurvedic medicines are traditionally prepared with mantras which serve to energize them on a subtle level. In addition, ayurvedic therapies are traditionally given along with the chanting of mantras. Along with Ayurveda, one should learn the basics of the Sanskrit language and the science of mantra so as to be able to benefit from this side of the teachings.

Ayurveda recommends bhakti yoga or devotion as one of the main tools of healing the heart. All those who seriously aspire to understand Ayurveda must recognize the supreme power of devotion and divine love for all deeper healing. In this regard, ayurvedic people should have a chosen form of God to worship that reflects their own devotion and faith in divine healing. This can be *Dhanvantari*, the deity of ayurvedic medicine who is a form of Vishnu, but it can be any of the names and forms of God or great teachers of humanity. Ganesha is also popular among ayurvedic practitioners. Many others prefer forms of the Divine Mother.

Ayurveda recommends jnana yoga or the yoga of knowledge for healing the mind, which requires meditation. Ayurveda is self-healing, which is only possible through self-knowledge. Ayurvedic students should use Ayurveda as a tool of self-examination even if this requires painfully examining our own errors and limitations.

Of course, an ayurvedic practitioner cannot be expected to

be proficient in all these yogas, but he or she must at least be aware of them and be capable of directing people to teachers who can help them along these paths. Only a great ayurvedic master will know all these yogas and be a doctor not only of the body but the mind and soul as well.

Yoga, too, should include Ayurveda in order to be complete. Hatha yoga is incomplete without an ayurvedic view of the body. Raja Yoga is incomplete without an ayurvedic understanding of the mind. All yogis must recognize the importance and value of right diet and herbs as yogic tools, and of ayurvedic purification measures like pancha karma as tools to prepare the body for yoga.

Generally, however, Ayurveda works at healing and purifying the body and mind while yoga aims at taking us to Self-realization, which depends upon a purified body and mind. In this way, the foundation of yoga should be Ayurveda and the fruit of Ayurveda should be yoga.

PART TWO

The Energetics of Yoga and Ayurveda

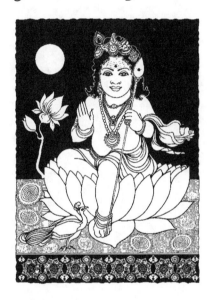

Secrets of Self-Transformation

6

The Soul and Its Different Bodies

The three — body, mind and soul — are like a tripod.
The world stands by their combination;
in them everything abides.
This combination exists for the
sake of the Purusha or conscious being.
It is the subject matter of Ayurveda for which the
teachings of Ayurveda have been revealed.

CHARAKA SAMHITA, SUTRASTHANA I.46-47

The human being is not simply a physical body, but a collection of three bodies that constitute various densities of matter, from the gross elements to most subtle layers of the mind. Behind these bodies resides our true Self that is beyond all manifestation, mental or physical. The three bodies, therefore, are not bodies in the ordinary sense but rather different types of encasements for the soul.

When yoga and Ayurveda address the human being and its needs, they are referring to this greater human being of the three bodies, not merely to the physical self, which in itself is little more than a collection of flesh and bones. Nor are they mainly addressing the higher Self or pure consciousness beyond all embodiment because that is not subject to suffering or ignorance and therefore does not need any help. Yoga and Ayurveda seek to unfold the mysteries of the subtle and causal bodies which serve as bridges to this higher Self. Without the development of these inner vestures, it is not possible to reach the divinity within us or to find real wholeness.

In this chapter we will discuss these three bodies along with their related five sheaths. This greater yoga and ayurvedic science of the three bodies and five sheaths[13] is the main concern of the book and the greater field of these two disciplines. The book aims at this original integral Yoga-Ayurveda, through which we can understand not only these two great systems and their interrelationship on all levels but also our greater being and function in the universe.

1. The Causal Body — the Magnetic Sphere of the Soul

The term soul refers to our deeper identity in life, which different thinkers define variously. In the Vedic sense, the soul means the reincarnating entity behind the veils of body and mind that endures throughout all our different births. This is called *jiva* in Sanskrit, meaning the "life power," or *jivatman*, Jiva-Atman, meaning the "individual Self or embodied soul," which is contrasted with *paramatman*, the "Supreme Self" or God beyond manifestation.

The jiva or soul is the basic unit or monad of creation. It is the ultimate indivisible entity or atom, the building block behind all matter in the universe, gross or subtle. All creation arises through the soul which is the causative power behind the cosmic manifestation. Our own soul itself is a divine creative power and our various lives are its creative play, its dreams or meditations. The soul is the divine flame or spark that descends into matter in order to fashion the worlds, creating structure, form and life. It contains direct knowledge of all our births, remaining in intimate contact with the divine, working as a servant to unfold the Divine Will.

The soul is not limited merely to human beings. It exists in all nature. Not only animals but also plants have a soul. The soul is hidden even in the rocks. However, the soul is not individualized in all creatures. In less-evolved forms it upholds their existence from behind. The soul also exists in advanced forms beyond humanity, as in gods, seers and angels. It can exist in darker creatures, anti-gods (*asuras*), but negative life forms do not always have a soul and can simply be figments of our imagination.

The soul directs all activities in the universe as the natural intelligence responsible for the marvelous order of creation. It plays behind the great forces of the earth, atmosphere, sky and stars. Universal soul forces work through the elements and uphold the laws of nature. An Earth soul sustains all life on the planet. Atmospheric, solar and planetary souls function as the guiding spirits or *devatas* behind the world process. The soul itself is like a sun, a source of light. Each individual contains such a secret sun in its heart as the soul force behind its being.

The soul is primarily a force of will and motivation, a seeking to do or become which reflects its creative power. Through the soul arise the various desires and aspirations that direct our karma. As a force of will, the soul possesses a magnetic energy that draws to us whatever we truly wish in our hearts. This magnetism of the soul holds together the different parts of our being and keeps them connected. It generates the energy that sustains the body and mind along with their different systems and faculties.

The World Soul similarly holds the world together, sustaining the various energies and processes of creation from the elemental realm to the kingdoms of the higher mind. The soul's

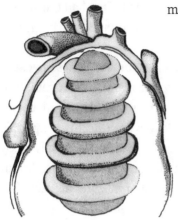

THE SPIRITUAL HEART

magnetism is responsible for the organic harmony not only of our own being, but of all creatures. This special magnetism of the soul exists on a deep level of consciousness beyond the ordinary mind and senses, maintaining our existence even in sleep and death.

The soul dwells within the hearts of all creatures, which is the source of real feeling and knowing. Yet this is not the physical heart but the core of our being, which we experience in the heart region of the physical body. The magnetic force of the soul, working through our hearts, holds us at a level that no external disturbance can reach. It regulates the heartbeat of creation. The causal body or sphere of the soul exists like a golden egg in the heart.[14]

The Three Powers of the Soul

The soul possesses three basic powers — life (*jiva*), light (*jyoti*), and love (*prema*) — from which arise the ability to perceive, move and feel. The soul's will is threefold: the will to be, the will to see, and the will to be happy. The magnetic force of the soul generates life, love and consciousness. From these three powers of the soul all creatures have three innate desires: to live forever, to know the absolute truth, and to feel perfect happiness. The arising of these aspirations shows the soul awakening within us.

The soul's magnetism is first of all a power of life, a

magnetic power that connects us with life and makes us feel alive, allowing us to move and breathe. Life is a current of energy that is generated by the magnetic force of the soul. Second, the soul's magnetism is a power of light, insight, wisdom and understanding. Light attracts and magnetizes our minds to it, just as all creatures are drawn to the sun. The soul possesses a power of illumination. Its nature is pure light. It is our inner sun that illumines the mind and senses. Its magnetism has a gravitational force, just as the gravitational force that comes from the sun.

Third, the soul's magnetic force is a power of love. It compels us to love all creatures and to love life. Love, after all, is the most powerful magnetic force of creation. It is the very power of attraction. Nothing else serves so strongly to bring creatures together and unite them at a core or heart level.

These three powers of life, light and love are the soul's reflection of Being-Consciousness-Bliss (*Sat-Chit-Ananda*), the threefold Godhead or Absolute. From them arise energy, light and matter as the main forces in the physical world. They give rise to the three great vital forces of *prana*, *tejas* and *ojas*, vitality, valor and endurance. They are behind the three active elements of air, fire and water, and the three doshas of vata, pitta and kapha.

THE THREEFOLD ORDER OF THE SOUL

Being	Consciousness	Bliss
Life	Light	Love
Prana	Tejas	Ojas
Air	Fire	Water
Vata	Pitta	Kapha

Charisma and Power of Character

Each soul projects a magnetic force according to its level of development. We can observe the soul's magnetism in our human interactions. We speak of magnetic personalities who have the power to draw people to them. Such individuals usually have a strong force of personality. However, this personality force is not always from the soul. It can be a thing of persuasion, sex, or manipulation. There are several levels and aspects of personal magnetism. Only the awakened soul, aware of its divine mission of Self-realization, has an entirely wholesome magnetic force. An unevolved soul can generate a strong ego energy, particularly if it has some mass following, which has its own sort of magnetism.

We all gravitate toward that with which our soul has affinity. This is owing to the magnetic nature of the soul. We draw to us people and circumstances that are in harmony with our soul and the type of manifestation that it is seeking. As we evolve spiritually, the Godward magnetized soul draws to itself divine influences — deities, teachers or experiences — to aid in its inner unfoldment. Our soul's magnetism, which is its power of love, brings us into various relationships and links us with other souls who further our soul quality and help us grow. This power of soul magnetism is the basis of the yogic emphasis on the *guru* (spiritual teacher) and *satsanga* (communion with the wise). Yet sometimes the soul draws us to people or situations that test it and challenge its growth as well, just as an advanced mountain climber will seek difficult slopes to climb.

Therefore, association is the main factor that magnetizes the soul. There is a entire science of association and personal magnetism known to yogis. The people we are drawn to in life reflect the nature of our soul's magnetism. So, too, the people we associate with in life hold our soul under their magnetic influences, which can either be hypnotic or enlightening. For this reason, yoga emphasizes right association as the foundation of yogic practice. Ayurveda similarly emphasizes right relationship as the basis of health. Unless we bring harmony into our relationships, the root of health and spiritual growth within us remains impaired. Wrong relationships not only cause emotional unrest but lead to improper actions with the body, mind and senses. After all, what we do and even what we eat reflects those with whom we associate.

If you want to understand the nature of your soul and its level of development, examine your relationships, not only physical ties but the people you emulate at a heart level and who function as your role models. The soul is reflected not so much by what we know but in the strength of our character, which is sustained by the people we look up to. The integrity of character projects the highest magnetic force that serves to integrate not only our own being but those of others.

The Magnetic Forces of the Knowledge and Ignorance

The magnetic force from the Creator determines the universal manifestation. Like all magnetic forces, it has a dualistic nature or polarity. There is both a cosmic force of attraction and one of repulsion. The attractive force has an internalizing or spiritualizing effect and elevates our consciousness. The repulsive force has an externalizing or materializing action and lowers consciousness. The attractive force promotes unity, healing and integration. The repulsive force causes conflict, disease and fragmentation.

The cosmic force of repulsion governs the descent of spirit into matter and creates the external world of names and forms. The cosmic force of attraction is the force of evolution that draws the embodied soul back to its divine Self and origin. These two forces are antithetical and mutually repulsive. The attractive or spiritual force repels the repulsive or worldly force. The repulsive or anti-spiritual force not only repels the divine but attracts unspiritual energies to itself. This force of repulsion to the divine and attraction to the external world is called *maya*, the power of illusion, or the power of ignorance (*avidya*). The force of divine attraction is called grace or Divine Shakti, the Divine Will (*Ishvara samkalpa*), or the power of knowledge (*vidya*).

The soul can be magnetized in one of these two directions. It can be drawn inwardly to divinity or externally to the outer world of enjoyment. It can be receptive to the magnetic force of divine attraction or that of divine repulsion, either moving toward the spirit or away from it. Divine attraction stimulates us to seek God or eternal truth. Divine repulsion creates attachment to external people and things, drawing us into transient involvement.

The force of divine attraction awakens our soul, making us conscious of ourselves as an immortal part of divinity seeking spiritual growth in the evolutionary cycle of rebirth. Divine repulsion creates the ego (*ahamkara*) or sense of our self as an outer or bodily identity, whose main goal is enjoyment in the external world. The force of divine repulsion or worldly attraction brings the soul into embodiment and causes it to seek happiness externally. This allows the outer forms and forces of the universe to be created. The force of divine attraction or detachment to the world then comes into play to complete the cycle of creation by drawing the soul back to its inherent divinity.

Both these magnetic currents are cosmic in nature and possess tremendous force. They are like two torrents, whose energy is irresistible. Whichever one we open ourselves up to will carry us along like a log upon a fast flowing stream. At the soul level we have only one basic choice: Which of these two types of magnetism should we become receptive to? Which of these two currents should we enter? Shall we function as spiritual beings seeking the unfoldment of consciousness in the universe or as egos, seeking our personal domination and enjoyment of outer reality?

We can observe to what degree our soul is magnetized to the divine or the undivine, to spiritual or worldly forces. We can see whether our love and attention is naturally directed internally to consciousness or externally to the world of form. We can see if our nature is to seek inner peace or outer enjoyment, inner expansion of awareness or outer expansion of possessions. As our present humanity is not very spiritually evolved, we will observe that most of us are caught in the current of ignorance and only have moments in which we are receptive to divine grace. However, we can cultivate this inner power and through it change the course of our lives. The inner current can overcome the outer current if we open ourselves up to the flow of grace.

The Three Gunas: The Magnetic Qualities of Nature

The magnetic force of maya or ignorance has three levels of operation, each of which has its characteristic quality and action. Our consciousness tends to get magnetized on one of these three levels. These are the three gunas of nature (*Prakriti*) of sattva, rajas and tamas, which are nature's three forces of knowledge, vitality, and embodiment.

Tamas is the darkest and heaviest magnetic density of ignorance. It draws to us forces of obstruction, decay and disintegration. It is the strongest force of the repulsive energy and serves to hold objects in form. Tamas inherently resists the divine will and is not receptive to any higher growth. We must let it go its own way until the shocks of life force it to change. Rajas is the middle density of ignorance. It creates illusions, fantasies, speculations, and imagination. It draws us into involvements, entanglements, complications and endless activity. The rajasic force can recognize the divine will, but distorts it according to its own ends. It can be turned into a spiritual force, but with difficulty and struggle.

Sattva is the subtlest density of nature and can reflect the power of divine attraction. It attracts what is refined and noble — the beauty of nature, art, philosophy, religion, service and charity. It possesses little resistance to the divine will but can remain outward in its orientation and get us caught in the external forms of goodness, if we do not direct it within. It easily becomes a spiritual force if used with knowledge, skill and detachment. Pure sattva (*shuddha sattva*), which is the inner form of sattva, develops the power of divinity. This is the one-pointed mind (*ekagra chitta*) of yogic thought.

Rajas and tamas make up the lower magnetic forces — the powers of cosmic repulsion that bind the soul to the external world. Tamas causes ignorance and rajas brings about attraction to the external world. The higher potentials for the gunas occur mainly through sattva, though it is possible for the divine will to work through higher forms of rajas and tamas as well.

The three gunas comprise the magnetic field for the soul. One guna usually predominates and polarizes our mind and life according to its qualities. Souls become either sattvic, rajasic or tamasic in nature. However, in the ordinary, unrefined field of human nature, one guna seldom prevails. After a time the other gunas must assert themselves. Our lives are an interplay of dullness, distraction and virtue, with shifting currents of good and evil, truth and falsehood.

Only a rare human being can become so totally dominated

by one guna that the other gunas lose their power. Such extreme types are the hardened criminal or complete tamasic type, the super achiever or complete rajasic type, and the selfless saint or complete sattvic type, but even these types can have their admixtures of the other gunas. Both Ayurveda and yoga seek to reduce the lower gunas of rajas and tamas. They are factors of mental and physical disease which Ayurveda addresses and the spiritual ignorance that yoga seeks to dispel.

The causal body or core mind is made up our deepest thoughts, desires, aspirations and intentions. These are called *samskaras* or *vasanas* in Sanskrit and are the magnetic imprints on our mindstuff, much like DNA holds the genetic code for the body. Samskara, meaning an imprint, refers to the seed motivations behind our behavior. Vasana, meaning a perfume, refers to how the deeper mind is shaped and colored by our moods and mental states. These tendencies hold the magnetic force that sustains our level of awareness. They reflect the gunas that we adhere to in life.

The higher spiritual magnetism or power of divine attraction makes up the soul force (*atma shakti*), which is the power of knowledge (*vidya shakti*). The lower or unspiritual magnetism, the power of divine repulsion, makes up the ego force or power of ignorance (*maya* or *avidya shakti*). The soul force is the power behind the development of true character and personality. The ego force is a power of personality without character. The soul force is developed through honesty, truthfulness and other ethical virtues, particularly through receptivity and caring for others. It cannot be developed through mere wishful thinking, emotional highs, or temporary experiences. It is the product of our daily action, particularly our most frequent thoughts and expressions. To function from the level of the soul in our human interactions is indeed difficult, though very rewarding if we make the effort.

Yoga, Ayurveda and the Soul

Yoga as a spiritual practice is only possible for the soul, for a person who has awakened his or her spiritual aspiration and longs to go beyond the cycle of rebirth. Yoga as spiritual practice is not possible for the unawakened or immature ego, which will use it for purposes of self-aggrandizement or personal enjoyment. To awaken at the level of the soul is the first step of genuine yoga practice and precedes even the yamas and niyamas, which require a soul awareness to be able to practice. If you wish to practice yoga, you must ask yourself: "Is the soul awake within me and ready to return to divinity?"

Ayurvedic healing is based upon our connection with the soul that is the origin of life and the energizing force behind all our faculties. Ayurveda works through the soul force so that we can master our physical body and integrate all our faculties to gain harmony and balance. All true healing comes from the soul, the conscious being within, which when awakened becomes a channel for divine grace.

2. The Subtle or Electrical Body

Out of magnetism, electricity automatically arises. The magnetic polarization or charge of the soul sets forth electrical currents and draws other currents to it from the external world. Out of the soul or heart arises the various electricities that sustain activity on all levels of our nature. The soul generates the force that creates and motivates the mind, senses and body. This electrical force is called *vidyut shakti*, literally "lightning" in Sanskrit. The magnetic sphere of the soul gives rise to an electrical field that creates the subtle or astral body, the sphere of our life energies and senses.

The two basic polar energies of the soul give rise the two basic pranas — Prana and Apana — which create attraction and repulsion, inhalation and exhalation, eating and elimination. These two pranas generate an electrical force that divides itself fivefold as the five pranas:

- *prana*, which moves inward,
- *apana*, which moves outward and downward,
- *samana*, which has a balancing action,
- *vyana*, which has an expansive action, and
- *udana*, which moves upward.

The five pranas, by their interaction with the mind, give rise to the five sense organs (ear, skin, eye, tongue, nose), five motor organs (speech, hands, feet, urinogenital, excretory) and five types of impressions (sound, touch, sight, taste and smell). These factors have already been noted in the scheme of cosmic evolution, the tattvas of the Samkhya system. The five pranas will be discussed in detail in the chapter on prana.

These electrical forces can function relative to any of the five magnetic levels of soul consciousness, from tamas to pure sattva. For example, our senses function at the level of tamas when they are dull and heavy. On the level of rajas, they draw us to distraction and involvement. On the level of ordinary sattva, they serve as instruments of knowledge and self-development. On the level of pure sattva, they function as powers of insight. On the transcendent level, they are withdrawn into inner powers of knowing.

On the lower levels, these electric forces work at low frequencies. Their action is slow and they make very few connections. On a higher level, their frequency rate increases. They make many connections and can penetrate eventually through all the levels of the universe of mind and matter. A true yogi experiences these forces in his own consciousness like perpetual lightning reverberating in all directions. This shows their full development.

This electrical body is called the subtle body because it is a vesture of energy more refined than physical matter. It is called the astral body because it is a field of light, the auric field of the mind and senses. Yet because its light is reflected from the soul, which is like the sun, it is called the lunar body. The subtle body is built up from the essence of energy and impressions, the pranas and tanmatras, which are the electrical forces that it brings into itself. As an electrical field it is highly active, moving and ever changing, dancing with all the fluctuations of the sense organs, motor organs and mind that are never restful even for a second.

The subtle body has a form similar to that of the physical body which it creates, but it exists more as an impression than as a specific object. The subtle body energizes and vitalizes the physical body, which it encompasses through the nervous and respiratory systems. All physical diseases have their origins in energy imbalances in the subtle body and its life-force. Ayurveda works to promote the healing powers of the subtle body, particularly its different pranas, to regenerate the physical body that arises from it. Yoga works to spiritualize the subtle body to turn it into a vehicle of spiritual realization.

Interrelationship Between the Causal and Subtle Bodies

Both subtle and causal bodies are different aspects of the entity that we usually call the mind, which has more levels and powers than what we ordinarily experience even in a highly intellectual life. The causal body is the deeper, subliminal or interior mind, beyond form and sensation, while the subtle body is the formal aspect of the mind, the outer layer of which constitutes our ordinary externally-directed sensory mentality.

The awakened or consciously functioning causal body is the field of superconsciousness beyond form, a purely ideal field of perception. The awakened subtle body is the field of superconsciousness within form — the realm of pure form, beauty and delight.

The casual and subtle bodies are closely related and are sometimes spoken of as one body.[15] The causal body endures throughout the entire cycle of rebirth. It undergoes an evolution to Self-realization but in itself is not born and does not die. A new subtle body is manifested out of the causal body with each birth and becomes the basis for the physical body, entering it in the womb.

The causal body therefore is the seed or unmanifest form of the subtle body. The subtle body is the manifest form of the causal body. All the potentials of the subtle body are inherent in the causal body. Like a turtle that puts forth its limbs from its shell, the causal body unfolds the astral body.

3. The Physical or Elemental Body

The causal body generates magnetic energy that gives rise to the electric force of the subtle body. This in turn creates a kind of rain that densifies as the gross or physical body. The electric force of the subtle body becomes the life force in the physical body. The magnetic force of the causal body becomes the indwelling consciousness or soul. The physical body, by its density, obstructs both the light and magnetism of the causal body and the electrical force of the subtle body. Its obstruction to the causal body, which is more refined, is greater than that of the subtle body. Yet these obstructions can be overcome by purification of the body and development of higher awareness through yogic practices.

The physical body develops from the subtle and causal bodies. The causal body provides the basic pattern and laws for it to follow. The genetic code, the magnetic imprint behind the physical body, is connected to the causal body. The subtle body's mind, prana, sense and motor organs shape the corresponding faculties of the physical body. The physical body encases the mind, senses and pranas in the denser medium of the bodily tissues.

The body is a creation of the gross elements. It is dominated by the doshas or biological humors of vata, pitta and kapha which are manifestations of prana at a gross level. Ayurveda describes the physical body according to its tissues, systems and organs. However, to change the physical body on a fundamental level, we must change the forces that produce it, its energetic electricity or astral background, and its magnetic imprint or causal basis. This is also the key to rejuvenation.

The Three States of the Soul: Waking, Dream and Deep Sleep

The three bodies relate to the three states of consciousness of waking, dream and deep sleep. The physical body functions during the waking state, in which we live in a world of physical objects with specific form and location in time and space. For this body to exist, we must take in the gross elements that compose it and which link us to the form world. Without the continual support of food, the gross body perishes.

The astral body functions during dream and inspired thought, in which we live in a world of our impressions. It defines time and space rather than being defined by them, as is the case with the physical body. It is sustained by impressions, the subtle elements which are its food, through which we create an internal world of our own imagination.

The causal body functions during deep sleep and profound meditation, during which we live in our own consciousness devoid of external objects, perceived or imaginary. The causal body is not located as a form or an impression in space and time, but exists as idea that creates time and space according to its qualities. It is sustained by our deeper thoughts and perceptions, the causal elements which are its food, through which we create a world of our own ideals.

These three states of consciousness reflect the process of death and rebirth. At death the physical body is withdrawn and the astral body comes into function just as in sleep and dream. The prana or life-force leaves the physical body and starts to function in the astral. The impressions gathered in life get revealed and through them one experiences happy or unhappy astral states, which in their extreme forms can become heavens and hells. Once these impressions are released, the astral body is withdrawn and the causal body comes into function. Prana and intelligence withdraw from the astral body and take one into the causal realm. The deeper qualities — the love and wisdom that one has gathered in life — are revealed and through them one experiences causal states, which are formless states of awareness. Once these are exhausted, then, from the causal body, new astral and physical bodies are set forth for another incarnation based upon the fructifying karma.

The Five Sheaths

The physical, astral and causal bodies make up five sheaths or layers of matter, with one intermediate sheath existing between the physical and astral bodies, and another between the physical and the causal. The three main functions of the mind constitute the three most subtle sheaths. Our inmost feelings, what is called *chitta* in yogic thought, make up the bliss sheath, the love at the core of our being. This is also the foundation of the mind or its inner aspect. Intelligence, the buddhi of yogic

THE THREE BODIES

	Gross or Physical Body	Subtle or Astral Body	Causal Body	Transcendant – Self or Pure Consciousness
Energetic Quality	Elemental	Electrical	Magnetism in action	pure magnetism
Light Quality	Heat	Lightning	light in manifestation	pure light
Composition	gross elements derived from food	Subtle elements derived from impressions	causal elements derived from gunas	consciousness only
State	Waking	Dream	deep sleep	turiya or transcendant
Existence	Physical	Astral	causal or ideal	unborn
Guna	Tamas	Rajas	Sattva	beyond gunas
Consciousness	ego or body identity	outer or sensory mind	inner mind or soul (Jiva)	Absolute

THE FIVE SHEATHS

Sphere	Sheath	Function	Composition	Symbol
Individualized Consciousness & Inner Mind/Chitta/Jiva	Anandamaya Kosha	Love and faith & intuitive feeling	Samskaras & gunas	Space
Intelligence/Buddhi	Vijnanamaya Kosha	Reason, discrimination & value-judgments	Intelligence & reason	Sun
Outer Mind & Senses/Manas	Manomaya Kosha	Sensory perception, knowledge of the external world	mind & five sense organs	Moon
Vital Force/Prana	Pranamaya Kosha	Energization of body & mind	five pranas & five motor organs	Wind
Gross Elements Physical Body	Annamaya Kosha	Sustaining embodied existence	five elements	Earth

thought, our capacity for judgment, makes up the intelligence sheath. The outer or sensory mind, called *manas*, and its emotions constitute the emotional sheath.[16]

Annamaya kosha is the physical body; it is composed of food but also contains the reflection of the other koshas upon it: pranamaya kosha through the circulatory/respiratory system; manomaya kosha through the nervous system and senses; vijnanamaya kosha through the brain; and anandamaya kosha through the reproductive system.

The pranic sheath is dual in nature. Its lower aspect becomes the physical pranas on the level of annamaya kosha, which generate life in the physical body, including the doshas. Its higher aspect generates the subtle pranas, those of manomaya kosha or outer mind. Pranamaya kosha itself is the sphere of the manifest pranas or vital energies which envelop the physical body and energize the mind through the senses. The pranic sheath in its outer aspect makes the physical body, which is otherwise a mass of flesh, come alive with sense and motor organs. Through its inner aspect, which is otherwise an expanse of space, it is able to manifest and express itself through the sense and motor organs.

Yet prana has even more subtle actions than the pranamaya kosha, which is only its sphere of manifestation. A seed prana exists on the causal level (anandamaya and vijnanamaya koshas) as the energy of the deeper mind and soul. In fact, the highest form of prana or vitality is *ananda* or bliss.

The intelligence sheath (vijnanamaya kosha) is dual in nature as well. Intellect, its lower function or discrimination directed toward the outer world, allows us to organize our impressions into fields of knowledge. This works along with the senses as part of the astral body and manomaya kosha. Its higher function is true intelligence or discrimination directed towards the eternal. This puts us in contact with universal law or dharma. It is part of the causal body (anandamaya kosha) and transcends the senses. The bliss aspect of buddhi or intelligence, the happiness and peace that comes through knowledge, functions through anandamaya kosha. Through the five sheaths we can understand the three bodies with more specificity.

7

Prana, Tejas and Ojas

Secrets of Yogic Alchemy

You are the ancient born Rishi, the one ruler
of the universe through the power of Ojas.

RIG VEDA VIII.6.41

Yoga is an alchemical process of balancing and transform
ing the energies of the psyche. To approach it we must
understand how to work with these energies in a practical
way. In this chapter we will introduce a deeper level of the
doshas that is important relative to yogic practice. Vata, pitta and
kapha have subtle counterparts called prana, tejas and ojas, which
could be called "the three vital essences." These are the root or
master forms of vata, pitta and kapha that control ordinary psychophysical functioning and, if reoriented properly, energize higher
spiritual potentials as well. They are not simply forces of the
physical body but of the subtle and causal bodies as well.

Prana, tejas and ojas are the essential or beneficial forms of
vata, pitta and kapha that sustain positive vitality. Unlike the
doshas, which are factors of disease, they promote health, creativity and well-being and provide the support for deeper yogic
and meditational practices.

Prana — primal life-force: the subtle energy of air as the master
force and guiding intelligence behind all psychophysical func-

87

tions, responsible for coordination of breath, senses and mind. On an inner level, it governs the unfoldment and harmonization of all higher states of consciousness.

Tejas — inner radiance: the subtle energy of fire as the radiance of vitality through which we digest air, impressions and thoughts. On an inner level, it governs the unfoldment of all higher perceptual capacities.

Ojas — primal vigor: the subtle energy of water as the stored-up vital reserve, the basis for physical and mental endurance; the internalized essence of digested food, water, air, impressions and thought. On an inner level, it is responsible for nourishing and grounding the development of all higher faculties.

These three forces are interrelated. Prana and tejas are rooted in ojas and can be regarded as aspects of ojas. Tejas is the heat and light energy of ojas that has an oily quality and, like ghee, can sustain a flame. Prana is the energy and strength that comes from ojas after it has been kindled into tejas. Ojas proper is the potential, the stamina of the mind and nervous system for holding tejas and prana. Ojas has the capacity to turn into tejas (heat), which has the capacity to turn into prana (electricity).

Prana, tejas and ojas resemble the concepts of *chi*, the Yang and Yin of Chinese medicine. Prana, as the life-force and cosmic breath, is like the primordial chi, which also relates to wind and spirit. Tejas as the power of will and vigor resembles original Yang, which is the primal fire. Ojas, as endurance and stamina, resembles primordial Yin, which is the essence of water.

The main rule of ayurvedic treatment is to prevent any of the doshas from becoming too high because in excess they cause disease. The dosha predominant in our constitution tends toward excess and must be restrained through the appropriate lifestyle regimen. This is achieved through following the right diet, herbs, exercise, and meditation that counter doshic proclivities.

In the practice of yoga a new rule comes into play. The yogi seeks to increase all three forces of prana, tejas and ojas. As these are the purified forms of the doshas, they do not have the same disease-causing power. These three vital essences only cause problems if one is increased at the expense of the others. They are basically wholesome energies that aid in renewal and transformation. The question is how to keep them growing at a similar rate so that their imbalance does not cause problems.

Increased prana is necessary to provide the enthusiasm, creativity and adaptability necessary for the spiritual path, without which we lack the energy and motivation to do our practices. Increased tejas provides the courage, fearlessness, and insight to take us along the path, without which we make wrong choices and judgments or fail to be decisive in what we do. Increased ojas is necessary for the peace, confidence and patience to keep our development consistent, without which we lack steadiness and calm. Should any of these factors be insufficient, our spiritual growth will be limited. These same factors increase positive health in both body and mind, and are helpful in treating all diseases, particularly of a chronic nature, including promoting rejuvenation.[17]

Functions of Prana, Tejas and Ojas

To understand these three forces let us examine how they function in the different aspects of our nature.

Reproductive System

Prana, tejas and ojas are nourished by the reproductive fluid which functions as their support in the physical body. They are three aspects of the transformed reproductive fluid (*shukra*). Ojas is the latent state of the reproductive fluid that provides not only reproductive power but strength in general and nourishes all the bodily tissues from within, particularly the nerve tissue. Ojas is our power of endurance and ability to sustain us, not only sexually but through all forms of exertion, physical and mental.

Tejas is the activated state of the reproductive fluid when it is transformed into heat, passion and will power. This occurs not only in sexual activity but whenever we are challenged or need to exert ourselves. Tejas gives us valor, courage and daring. In yoga this force is necessary to enable us to perform tapas or transformative spiritual practices. Prana is the life-creating capacity inherent in the reproductive fluid. This aids in longevity and rejuvenation and stimulates the flow of prana through the nadis, giving a deeper energy to the mind. Without the proper reserve of reproductive fluid, we will become deficient in prana, tejas and ojas. Wrong or excessive sexual activity depletes all three forces.

Endocrine System

Prana, tejas and ojas relate to the endocrine system. Prana governs equilibrium, adaptability, and growth processes. The pineal and pituitary glands, which are the master controllers of growth and intelligence, are prana predominant. This is why most disorders in the growth process, like in people who are unusually tall or short, are generally vata (air) problems.

Tejas governs metabolism and digestion. Thyroid and pancreas functions are tejas predominant. Most deep-seated metabolic problems are tejas in nature. Ojas governs reproduction and energy reserve and dominates in the testes, ovaries and adrenals. Most problems of the reproductive system are ojas related. Ojas also allows us to handle stress through sustaining adrenaline.

Immune System

Prana, tejas and ojas give energy to the immune system. Ojas is the basic capacity of the immune system, our potential to defend ourselves against external pathogens. It provides endurance, resistance and strength to ward off diseases.

Tejas is the immune system which is able to burn and destroy toxins when activated. It generates the fever that the body produces to destroy the pathogens which attack it. Tejas is our ability to overcome acute diseases, which are generally infectious in nature. Tejas is ojas converted into heat, warmth and vitality. It is our ability to mobilize our immune system's forces.

Prana is the long-term activation of the immune function to project and develop life-energy, which manifests when we are dealing with a chronic disease. It is the adaptability of the immune system and sustains all long-term healing processes. With sufficient prana, tejas and ojas, no disease can approach us. Increasing prana, tejas and ojas helps all low immune conditions.

Nervous System and Nadis

The nervous system is the master system governing all bodily systems. The three vital essences are responsible for its proper function. Prana governs the discharge and coordination of nerve impulses, which are pranic and vata forces. When deranged, it causes hypersensitivity, tremors and imbalances in the nervous system. Tejas provides acuity of perception and feeling. Deranged tejas burns out the nervous system, causing inflammation and scarring of the nerve tissue. Ojas gives endurance and stability through the nervous system. It is responsible for the lubrication of the nerve channels. Nervous breakdown or nervous exhaustion occurs through low ojas.

Prana, tejas and ojas govern the movement of impulses through the nadis as well. Ojas is the fluid that lines the nadis, cushioning the flow of energy through them. Tejas is the heat moving through them. Prana is the energy moving produced by the heat of tejas. To safeguard the nadis we must protect prana, tejas and ojas.

Breath

The three vital energies are closely connected to the breath through the pranamaya kosha. Prana is the basic energy and movement of the breath, its propulsive source and power of action. Tejas is the heat produced by the breath, including its ability to vitalize the blood. Ojas is the deeper energy that we absorb through the breath and store at a deep level of the heart and solar plexus.

When prana is deranged, the breath becomes shallow or disturbed. When tejas is deranged, the heat content of the breath is abnormal. When ojas is deranged, the absorbed energy of the breath is low. We are unable to hold and consolidate prana. Those practicing pranayama should maintain a close examination of the condition of their prana, tejas and ojas.

Senses

Prana, tejas and ojas as powers of the mind function through the senses. Prana allows for the equilibrium and coordination of sensory impulses and is predominant in the ears (including the inner ear) and the skin, the vata-predominant (ether and air) senses. Tejas is responsible for acuity of sensory function and our ability to digest sensory impressions. It dominates in the eyes, the pitta or fire-predominant sense. Ojas is responsible for stability of the senses, as well as for their lubrication. It dominates in the tongue and the nose, the kapha-predominant (water and earth) senses.

Creativity

On an inner level, prana, tejas and ojas are measures of creativity. Ojas is latent creative capacity, our storehouse of creative energy. Tejas is creative vision, the ability to see new things and break with the past. Prana is creative action to bring new things into being and remain in the creative state. Proper ojas is necessary to give us a good reserve of creative energy to draw upon. Proper tejas serves to direct our creative energy toward specific goals and projects. Proper prana functions to keep our creativity mobile and transformative. Without sufficient prana, tejas and ojas, we are unable to make positive changes in our lives.

Mind and Soul

Prana, tejas and ojas exist on deeper levels of the mind and soul. The pranic force behind the mind allows it to move and respond, providing its basic energy. The tejas force of the mind allows it to perceive and to determine, giving it light and heat. The ojas force of the mind gives it patience, consistency and steadiness in the application of attention.

Each sustains certain emotions. Prana gives emotional harmony, balance, enthusiasm and joy. Tejas gives courage, fearlessness, and daring that allows us to accomplish heroic or extraordinary actions. Ojas provides emotional peace, love, calm and contentment. Without these emotional forces the mind remains unstable.

Similarly, there is a prana in our deeper consciousness that guides the soul throughout the entire process of incarnation, creating and energizing its various embodiments. The soul's tejas is its accumulated insight and wisdom, its flame of spiritual aspiration. The soul's ojas is the material through which it produces and sustains all of its various bodies. These higher forms of prana, tejas and ojas reside along with the soul in the spiritual heart, which is their ultimate point of origin and end. The *Vedas* often refer to the soul as prana or tejas.

Kundalini — Shakti Energy/ Amrit — Shiva Energy

Kundalini develops from all three — prana, tejas and ojas — but primarily tejas. As the inner fire, it is mainly the heightened energy of tejas carrying the awakened pranic force and sustained by a higher ojas. Kundalini as subtle fire is a form of lightning or electrical force on an inner level.

Kundalini as tejas is the higher feminine energy or yoga shakti, the power of yoga, necessary to catalyze all higher evolutionary potentials within us. Opposite to kundalini is the *amrit* or nectar that descends from the crown chakra and feeds the kundalini in her upward ascent. This is the purified ojas energy in the subtle body which has been extracted and distilled through spiritual practice. Ojas is the higher masculine or Shiva energy which, through surrender, care and protection, falls in a descent of grace. While some people experience the ascending fire, others experience more fully the descending nectar.

The union of tejas (kundalini) and ojas (amrit) creates the highest prana, which is the immortal life energy that the kundalini carries the way a mother carries her child. This alone has the power to create the higher samadhis necessary to dissolve the deep-seated conditionings in our consciousness that cause our attachment to the cycle of birth and death. This immortal prana is the divine child or child of immortality and derives from the higher tejas and ojas energies that it carries.

This higher prana is the power or shakti of our higher intelligence (buddhi), which enables us to discriminate between the eternal and the transient, the divine and the undivine, giving enlightenment to the soul. Without such a deep energy in the mind, whatever meditation we do and whatever insight we gain, we will be unable to hold or consolidate it.

Building Prana, Tejas and Ojas

Prana, tejas and ojas can be developed in several ways. We possess a certain amount of them congenitally, which is reflected in the inherent strength of our constitution, but they can be increased by various practices. They must first be purified (rendered sattvic) for their yogic affects to come forth. This requires a pure diet and dharmic living, along with control of the mind, emotions and senses such as yoga ordinarily prescribes. In other words, yogic living is the foundation to work with them.

Increasing Ojas

Ojas increases in several ways, of which the following are most important:

1) Right Diet
2) Tonic Herbs
3) Control of Sexual Energy
4) Control of the Senses
5) Devotion (Bhakti Yoga)

Right Diet

Ojas, as a subtle material substance and essence of the tissues, requires the material support of a right diet. This involves a nutritive vegetarian diet with the use of whole grains, seeds and nuts, oils, root vegetables and natural sugars. A cruder form of ojas can be developed through animal products but this is too heavy to be of any value for the spiritual path. The sattvic diet outlined in the section on diet can be followed, with emphasis on the nutritive side — whole grains, dairy products, seeds, nuts, oils and sweet fruit.

Tonic Herbs

Herbs for ojas are mainly tonic or nutritive in nature, having food value and rejuvenative (soma-producing) potentials, like ashwagandha or ginseng. They are usually taken along with food. Note the herbs to increase physical energy and vitality and to strengthen ojas in the section on herbs.

Brahmacharya

Control of sexual energy (brahmacharya) means reducing the discharge of reproductive fluid. This is crucial for developing additional ojas. It can be achieved by reducing one's sexual activity. To a lesser extent it can be done by having sex without orgasm, the type of practice taught both in tantric and Taoist sexual yogas. While sexual restraint is difficult for our modern sexually-oriented society, we cannot for that reason ignore its value in yoga. It is not a question of morality but of energy. If we discharge our sexual energy, which is the strongest energy of the body, we may not have enough fuel to carry us in our practices. But we must do this with spiritual aspiration to be really able to sublimate our energy. As mere repression it cannot take us very far.[18]

Control of the Senses

Control of the senses requires reducing the amount of energy lost through sensory indulgence, which includes avoiding most forms of entertainment, particularly through the mass media. Much energy is lost through the eyes and the ears. This is part of the practice of *pratyahara* or withdrawal from the senses in Raja Yoga. Overuse of the motor organs can also deplete ojas, particularly too much talking because the vocal organ is the most important of these. Overwork or overexertion of any type should be avoided when ojas is low.

Devotion

Devotion (bhakti yoga) is the best yogic path for developing ojas. This means redirecting our emotional energy inwardly through love of God in whatever form or relationship is dearest to us. Devotion helps us control our senses and our sexuality and transmutes animal emotions into more refined feelings. This can be done through various forms of devotional worship, rituals, prayers, repeating divine names, and service to God and guru. Note the section on bhakti yoga.

Increasing Tejas

Once ojas is sufficient, we can turn it into tejas without depleting it. Tejas is primarily developed through:

1) Control of speech and other austerities (tapas)

2) Mantra

3) Concentration exercises

4) Yoga of Knowledge (Jnana Yoga)

Control of Speech

Controlling speech means avoiding aimless talking and gossiping and also avoiding critical and abusive speech. Periods of silence are helpful, like not speaking one day a week or being silent in the evening. This helps develop an internal energy of insight and takes us more into a witnessing state. Other austerities, such as fasting or staying awake at night, are helpful in developing tejas because they increase our fire of determination.

Mantra

Mantra is a higher form of control of speech that develops the inner fire. The Goddess Kundalini is said to wear the garland of the letters of the Sanskrit alphabet around her neck. She is made up of mantra. There are many ways to use mantra. Repetition of the Sanskrit alphabet is one way. Repetition of certain *bija* (seed) mantras, particularly OM, HUM and HRIM, is another. Longer mantras like Gayatri are very good. Generally mantras should be first spoken out loud for a short period of time, then muttered with a low voice for a longer period, and then repeated on a purely mental level for a yet longer period. There are mantras useful for ojas and prana as well, like SHRIM for ojas and KRIM for prana.

Concentration Exercises

Concentration exercises (dharana) involve focusing the mind on a particular object, which may be outer like a flame, inner like visualization of the form of a deity, or an element, idea or truth principle. Concentration gives acuity of mind that causes our inner fire to come forth. Concentrating on the inner light perceived in the region of the third eye is an important method to develop tejas. Learning to direct our power of vision helps in this regard. Tejas is what allows the third eye to open.

Yoga of Knowledge

The yoga of knowledge (jnana yoga) is fire-predominant, particularly the practice of various forms of inquiry, like Self-inquiry. This consists of holding to the inquiry "Who am I?" and letting go of other thoughts. Tejas arises through the development of discrimination (*viveka*), which means discerning the eternal from the transient, the unchanging truth from changing names and forms. This is the main movement of our inner intelligence (buddhi) as it awakens in us as insight.

Increasing Prana

Once ojas and tejas are developed, a higher prana can come forth. Prana is developed specifically through pranayama, but many other methods are helpful:

1) Pranayama
2) Passive meditations emphasizing space and sound
3) Raja or Integral Yoga

Pranayama

Pranayama develops prana not only on an outer but also on an inner level. As the ingoing and outgoing breaths become balanced, we contact our inner prana. This we experience as a sense of lightness, expansion or ascension of energy. However, pranayama can be used for developing tejas and ojas as well and can aid in the integration of all three factors. Pranayama generates heat, particularly through retention of the breath, that increases tejas, which is related to the fire of the breath (*pranagni*). It helps transform the reproductive fluid and lower forms of ojas into a more spiritual form. Note chapters on prana and pranayama for how to do this.

Passive Meditation

Meditation on space or the void is another way to develop prana. Prana is born of space. Wherever space is created, prana must come into being. Creating inner space creates the inner prana automatically. Another method is to meditate upon the inner sounds, which arise from the inner space. The heart itself is the region of inner space and the ultimate source of sound. Meditation on sound and space in the heart connects us with the original power of prana.

Raja Yoga

Raja Yoga emphasizes using prana to calm the mind along with other techniques of mantra, concentration and meditation. Prana is the mobility and adaptability of consciousness brought about by employing various diverse methods of meditation. According to Raja Yoga, the *vrittis* or movements of the mind are controlled by prana. By prana we can control the mind.

Raja Yoga is an integral approach combining both the yoga of knowledge and the yoga of devotion. This also helps develop prana, which is born of the union of wisdom and devotion. In this regard, the practices mentioned under both ojas and tejas must be done together. For example, generally the yoga of knowledge is best done in the morning and the yoga of devotion in the evening.

Keeping Prana, Tejas and Ojas in Balance

As these three factors are always closely related, the practices help develop each other. An integral development of prana, tejas and ojas, therefore, is the key to a balanced inner growth. Of these the most important is ojas. Ojas not only gives a strong reserve of vital energy, it also provides strength and maturity of character and emotional stability. Ojas creates the vessel necessary to hold prana and tejas, which would otherwise disperse. One may have a very intelligent mind or sensitive heart but these will not take us far spiritually without the proper ojas or vital juice to support them. Without ojas, exercises in meditation and yoga lack the proper foundation. Perhaps the first question for an individual attempting real yogic practices is: "Do I have the ojas to sustain it?"

Prana is held by ojas, which is its conductor. If we increase prana without ojas, adding energy without being able to ground it, we may disturb, if not derange, the mind and nervous system. Tejas rests on ojas, which is its fuel. If we increase the critical capacity of the mind, our power of discrimination (tejas), without increasing ojas, we will literally burn ourselves up. Spiritual knowledge can only burn if fed with the fuel of love.

Once sufficient ojas is there, one needs to develop tejas in order to utilize it. This requires will, insight and discernment: choosing the right path and following it consistently. Then one can develop prana, which comes from the union of tejas and ojas. Once we have the right foundation and are taking the right path, prana allows us to move swiftly along the way.

Prana, Tejas and Ojas and Disease

Generally any excess of the doshas, whether vata, pitta or kapha, will eventually weaken all three forces of prana, tejas and ojas. The doshas when excessive also prevent their own higher or subtle forms from developing.

High vata dries up ojas as wind dries up water. It weakens tejas as wind agitates a fire or blows it out. However, high vata depletes prana as well. When vata is formed as a waste gas, the subtle energy of prana, which is like a rarefied fragrance, cannot form.

High pitta burns up ojas, as too high a flame consumes the oil that feeds it. It weakens prana in the same way that heat and fever exhaust our vitality. Yet high pitta also damages tejas. Pitta dosha is a crude form of tejas that cannot be converted into the subtle essence of tejas, just as oil that is filled with contaminants cannot produce a good flame. Let us take an example. Tejas is valor and courage. High pitta is anger and paranoia. When pitta is in excess, these higher qualities of tejas cannot manifest.

High tejas and prana can damage ojas but these are temporary because they are destroying their own root. Excess tejas is like a high fire that consumes its fuel and must eventually go out. This is like a soldier on a battlefield who pushes his courage until he loses it and turns into a coward. It is different from high pitta because exhaustion of ojas in this case is not caused by a toxin but by excessive use of a positive energy. Similarly, a person with a great deal of creative prana can exhaust their ojas by overwork. Young people in particular can have high levels of prana or tejas for some time before their ojas gets depleted. This is because they have a good congenital ojas to draw upon.

Deeper vitality disorders involve imbalances of prana, tejas and ojas, which affect the deeper bodily systems — the nervous and reproductive systems, the senses and the mind. These include growth disorders in children, premature aging, metabolic problems, hormone imbalances, nervous system problems, allergies, and most degenerative diseases from cancer to AIDS. When these subtle master energies are deranged, physical function is disturbed at a deep level with ramifications on all systems and organs. Psychological imbalances affect prana, tejas and ojas, which are closely connected to the senses, emotions and mind. These include anxiety, anger, depression, attachment and grief. By increasing prana, tejas and ojas, most psychological problems can be alleviated.

Most meditation disorders are caused by imbalanced development of prana, tejas and ojas. Their main cause is insufficient ojas. Without the proper ojas, increased tejas can burn up the nadis of the subtle body. This can occur from excessive practice of meditation or mantra without the proper ojas to sustain it. Without the proper ojas, increased prana can move in erratic ways. This can occur from excessive practice of pranayama or trying to empty the mind without having the proper ojas to support it. We should be careful in attempting powerful practices if our ojas is not sufficient.

Yoga is an alchemical process that requires knowledge of the forces that we are working with. It is not mere wishful thinking, nor does it occur only in the mind. The ayurvedic science of prana, tejas and ojas provides the understanding of the subtle forces of yoga. While it is a more complex matter than the synopsis given in this chapter, the reader should have a sense of the dynamics involved.

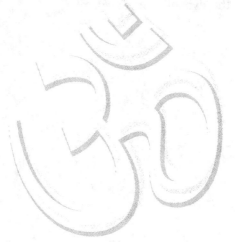

8

Agni Yoga

Harnessing the Inner Fire

He has no disease, nor old age, nor death, who has
attained a body born of the fire of Yoga.

SHVETASVATARA UPANISHAD II.12

Yoga is a ritual fire in which we offer our body, life and mind into the flame of awareness that is our true Self. This inner fire takes us across the dark night of ignorance to the perpetual day of enlightenment. A great yogi is a living flame whose very presence fills us with light, warmth and vitality.

The practice of yoga is all about creating the fire of yoga, which should be its foundation. Similarly, Ayurveda is a great fire offering. We must create the fire of healing to make ourselves well and to sustain positive health and vitality. An ayurvedic doctor should have the warmth of that cosmic flame of life.

This principle of fire in the universe is called *agni* in Sanskrit, meaning "the transforming force." It is not simply fire in the elemental sense but all potentials of heat, light and electricity. This divine fire is the origin of life, light and love — the powers of the soul that motivate us from within. The soul itself is our inner fire, the spiritual aspiration deep within us that accompanies us through all our births. It is the inextinguishable flame, the witness behind all our states of consciousness, the ever-wakeful seer. We are manifestations of this divine fire that is the Self of all.

Yoga and Ayurveda as Fire Rituals

Yoga and Ayurveda are both sciences of agni or the divine fire (*agni vidyas*). They teach us how the cosmic fire works so that through it we can achieve all necessary balance and growth. The cosmic fire that exists outwardly on all planes of the universe, from gross matter to pure being, has its counterpart within us on all layers of our individual nature, from the physical body to our immortal consciousness. It is the catalytic force necessary for any evolutionary change to occur. Ayurveda emphasizes the role of agni on a physical level and shows us how to balance our digestive fire as the basis of physical health. Yoga emphasizes the fires of prana and meditation as the means of enlightenment.

The Outer Fire Ritual

The *Vedas* teach an elaborate fire ritual called *yajna* or sacrifice. Yajna refers to a redirection or transformation of energy, a change of substance from one level to another. The idea behind the yajna is that whatever one offers to the divine must be transformed to a higher level of manifestation.

In the yajna a special fire is made according to a specific procedure. An altar or fire pit is constructed. Special wood is used as fuel and the fire is enkindled in a precise manner, preferably by the rubbing together of sticks. In this sacred fire we place various offerings, like rice or ghee, that both feed the fire and are transformed by it into various essences. Along with these offerings we recite various prayers and mantras, seeking to fulfill our wishes and bring divine blessings into the world.

The fire is the messenger between the material world and

higher spiritual realities, between man and the gods. What we offer in the fire is carried to the invisible realms where higher powers can recognize and act upon it, sending back their grace. Such a sacred fire serves to purify the environment, not only on a gross but on a subtle level. It works to purify the astral bodies of those who perform it regularly. Such a ritual should

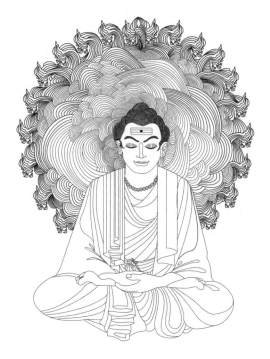

THE YOGI AS AGNI

be done in each home or ashram on a regular basis.

Fire offerings can be used to achieve the ordinary goals of life like health, wealth and prosperity. They can be done for inner purposes of working out difficult karma, propitiating negative planetary influences, or consecrating various spiritual practices. They are part of a universal technology of inner evolution.

The ashes of the fire, called *bhasma*, possess purifying, healing and curative powers. Sometimes special herbs go into their making. Such bhasmas can be used to potentize other medicines or are taken as a medicine themselves. Bhasmas made in the presence of great spiritual masters are particularly powerful.

The most important times for fire rituals are sunrise, noon and sunset offerings, called *agnihotra* or fire invocations. New and full moon offerings are also important and, in Vedic times, various seasonal and yearly offerings were performed as well. Such transitional or juncture points, called joints or *sandhis* in Sanskrit, are times at which energy naturally changes and can be more easily worked upon and redirected.

The Ayurvedic Fire Ritual

In the ayurvedic fire ritual, the fire is the digestive fire or *jatharagni*. The offerings are the food that we eat. This is called *pranagnihotra*, or the pranic fire offering, as taught in the *Vedas*. In this we offer our food not only to the jatharagni but to the five pranas that work with it.

Before eating we should first sprinkle some pure water around our food to purify it. One can simply chant OM while doing this or do the whole Gayatri mantra, if one knows it. Then one should chant: "You are the tablecloth of immortality, Swaha!"[19] and sip a little water. Then one should recite the mantras to the five pranas, at each time taking a little food in the mouth, remembering the prana and its action as a divine force that sustains us.

OM Pranaya Swaha!

OM Apanaya Swaha!

OM Vyanaya Swaha!

OM Samaya Swaha!

OM Udanaya Swaha!

Then one should finish the meal and recite: "You are the covering of immortality, Swaha!"[20] Swaha is the mantra for making any offerings to the sacred fire. In this way the food we eat nourishes all our pranas through the instrumentality of the digestive fire.

Yoga, the Inner Fire Ritual

Yoga is an inner fire ritual that does not use external ingredients but rather the different faculties of our nature. In the practice of yoga we offer all aspects of our being into the inner fire of God. There are different yogic fire rituals depending which faculties we offer. Yoga uses the fire of breath and mind to purify and transform our consciousness. This occurs by linking ourselves with the divine fire that is God or the inner Self. It requires awakening the fire of our soul to take us back to the god or divine sun within. Our subtle body and its system of nadis and chakras is like a great tree that needs to be lit up by the inner fire of kundalini which emanates from the soul. The yogi himself becomes fire, which opens his third eye and becomes a force that he can project upon the world. All true yogis seek to develop the yogic fire.

The Fires in the World of Nature

Many forms of agni exist in the world of nature and direct the process of evolution. First is the elemental fire that exists in the Earth and in the stars, which itself has many forms. Then there is the vegetable fire that produces organic life through photosynthesis. This gives rise to the animal fire that breeds emotion and passion. The animal fire deepens into the true human fire that promotes truth and compassion. This generates the angelic fire that enkindles love and devotion.

These five cosmic fires relate to the five koshas defined below. Highest is the atmic fire or fire of the Self that is pure consciousness, which is also the Brahmic fire or absolute flame of pure existence beyond these.

The Seven Agnis and the Five Koshas

Each of the five koshas or encasements of the soul has a different form of agni responsible for its development. Like the digestive fire, agni on all levels is the force of growth and balance, allowing nutrients to be taken in and waste materials to be eliminated.

1. Agni of the Food Sheath, Annamaya Kosha

The agni of the food sheath is the digestive fire (jatharagni) which dwells in the abdomen, particularly in the small intestine where the main digestion of food occurs. The digestive fire breaks down the food we eat into the essence of the five elements. From its action arises the digested food mass that provides nourishment to all the tissues through the plasma. Through it we digest food, which gets transformed into the tissues of the body.

The act of eating, taking the food into the mouth and the stomach, is kapha (water) predominant, requiring the liquefaction of the food. The action of digestion, breaking down and absorbing the food in the small intestine is the field of pitta (fire), with which agni is closely related. The action of elimination through the large intestine is in the field of vata (air), where the waste gases are held and released. So all three doshas can be worked upon through jatharagni.

The physical agni is closely linked with speech, which is the dominant action of the mouth. In fact, the physical body is a tube built around the digestive tract whose main opening is the mouth. Right eating and right speaking are complementary processes of the food sheath. One should take care not only what goes into the mouth but what comes out of it.

2. Agni of the Pranic Sheath, Pranamaya Kosha

The agni of the pranic sheath is *pranagni*, the agni of prana. It works in the lungs and heart and connects with the jatharagni in the solar plexus below, which is also the physical pranic center. Pranagni is responsible for converting oxygen from the external air into an internal force of vitality. Pranagni connects with the blood, serving both to oxygenate it and to give it a red color. Through pranagni we digest air or prana, which gets transformed into energy. The energy of the breath is more subtle and immediate than that of food.

The action of inhalation, like that of eating, is in the field of kapha and that of exhalation, like elimination, in the field of vata. Pranagni is energized through retention of the breath, which is connected with pitta. Pranagni is also connected with speech, particularly speech as energized with breath.

3. Agni of the Outer Mind, Manomaya Kosha

The agni of the outer mind is the fire of perception, *manasika agni*. This allows us to digest sensory impressions. Among the sense organs, the mental fire is most connected with the eye, which corresponds to fire among the senses. Among the motor organs it is most connected with speech on the mental level — the speech within the mind, our internal voice. The mental agni digests impressions and turns them into our inner landscape, the field of our imagination.

4. Agni of Intelligence, Vijnanamaya Kosha

The agni of intelligence is the fire of discrimination, through which we can discern truth and falsehood, good and bad, right and wrong. The fire of the outer mind is neutral morally. It simply digests impressions. The fire of intelligence digests these further, extracting their meaning, quality or content — their underlying idea. From it our basic values and beliefs are constructed. The agni of intelligence builds up the body of dharma, our field of insight and understanding.

5. Agni of Bliss, Anandamaya Kosha

The agni of this sheath is the fire of love, which in the undeveloped person is the fire of desire. This is the flame of our deepest wishes, motivations and aspirations. Desire can be transformed into the fire of divine love and bliss. This depends upon feeding our fire of bliss not with sensory enjoyments but with devotion to the divine. The agni of bliss takes in the feeling content of our experience and extracts delight out of it. This is the body of joy that wisdom allows to grow.

6. Self — Chidagni, the Fire of Consciousness

Consciousness itself has the nature of fire, light and illumination. It is also called the fire of knowledge, but in the higher sense as spiritual or Self-knowledge — the fire of consciousness (*Chidagni*) or the fire of awareness. This is the real inner fire or light from which all the other fires derive their light and energy by reflection. It is the seer of all and the entire universe is its body.

7. Brahman — The Fire of Brahman or Fire of Being

The fire of Brahman (*brahmagni*), which is the fire of being, and the fire of consciousness (chidagni) are not different, but two aspects of the same reality. Brahmagni is the fire of existence or universal fire. It is beyond all duality and is a self-consuming reality. All existence is a self-existent fire. This is the supreme reality.

The Five Agnis of the Koshas and Limbs of Yoga

Ayurveda is based upon the development of agni, mainly on a physical level, balancing the jatharagni for proper digestion of food and elimination of toxins. Yet it also works to improve pranagni, the fire of vitality, through herbs, exercise and special therapies like pancha karma, ayurvedic detoxification measures.

Yoga is more concerned with the development of agni on the higher levels, particularly as the fire of intelligence that connects with the divine fire or flame of awareness that is the Purusha. Through meditation and samadhi yoga, one develops the agnis of the higher koshas of intelligence and bliss. Yoga practice is meant to develop the fire of yoga in order for the process to work. Fire is the factor that brings about all ripening and transformation.

Yet in yoga the key agni is pranagni. There is a special connection between pranagni and all deeper agnis. Prana is the primary energy. Pranagni is the most powerful agni. It can purify the subtle body to allow for the inner experiences of yoga to come forth. Until that is developed, the higher aspects of yoga cannot unfold.

The practice of Raja Yoga and its eight limbs is designed to develop all five agnis to aid in our inner purification and transformation. The yamas and niyamas, the rules and disciplines of the yoga system, serve to put our outer life in order so we can prepare the fuel of our nature for its enkindling by the divine fire. Their practice serves to mature our character so that it can hold the inner fire. Unless the fuel, which is our mind and body, is prepared properly it cannot be burned by this inner power. Yogic disciplines of nonviolence, truthfulness, control of sexual energy, self-discipline, self-study and surrender to God function make the fire of our life glow more brilliantly and ripen our character for spiritual practice to be efficacious.[21]

Asana and Jatharagni

The practice of asana or yogic postures serves to balance, stabilize and further enkindle the jatharagni or physical agni, which helps purify the physical body. When the physical body is still, relaxed and balanced, the digestive fire is also balanced and purified. Correct performance of asana results in good digestion and elimination, a regular and healthy but not excessive appetite. Various postures aid in the increase of the digestive fire, particularly sitting poses and uddiyana bandha.

Pranayama and Pranagni

The main purpose of pranayama is to develop pranagni, the fire of the prana for purification of the prana, nadis and subtle body. Pranagni develops mainly between inhalation and exhalation. Pranagni, we might add, is a force different than the five pranas yet connected with all of them as their heat and electrical connection.

Pranayama, deep breathing combined with retention of the breath, increases pranagni. Pranagni increases body heat leading to sweating, which helps purify the nadis. The combination of pranayama and mantra aids in its development and in the purification of pranamaya kosha.

Pratyahara and the Agni of the Senses (Indriya Agni)

Pratyahara is literally fasting from sensory impressions, but includes all methods of control of the senses and motor organs, and the internalization of attention. This serves to increase the Agni of the outer mind and senses, through which we can detoxify the mind of negative impressions.

Dharana and the Agni of the Mind

The fire of the mind must burn steadily for it to be able to penetrate into the nature of reality. The mental fire burns steadily when it can consistently hold to a certain object of attention. This is the practice of dharana by which the fire of attention can grow in luster and strength.

Dhyana and the Agni of Intelligence

Meditation is the means of increasing our fire of intelligence. For this our thoughts are the fuel and the witness consciousness is the fire. By remaining in the state of the seer, all things become fuel for awareness.

Samadhi and the Agni of Love

Samadhi or spiritual absorption occurs when the object of our contemplation merges fully into the fire of contemplation. In this we must merge into the divine fire that burns within our hearts, which will purify us of all our outer desires. We enter the fire of bliss.

The Natural State of Samadhi and the Fire of Consciousness

The divine Self ever exists in the state of samadhi or spiritual oneness. This samadhi is a constant state, unlike the samadhis of the mind which are particularized and come and go as various levels of experience. The Self is the divine fire which is the eater of all. For it, all the universe is food. It can consume any experience, good or bad, true or false. This is the fire of being and consciousness beyond all multiplicity.

Keys to the Development of the Seven Agnis

1. Jatharagni — Digestive Fire

   • Right balance of food eaten and feces eliminated through right digestion and absorption.

   • Right diet according to constitution with sattvic food, proper oil like ghee in the diet to support agni. Regular eating habits with seasonal and stage-of-life variations.

   • Right spices like ginger, cardamom, turmeric, cayenne and black pepper.

   • Fasting to enkindle the digestive fire.

   • Physical calm and release of tension through asana and right exercise.

   • Regulation of body temperature and developing resistance to cold and temperature changes.

2. Pranagni - Fire of Prana

   • Breathing of good quality air, rich in prana.

   • Right balance of breath inhaled and breath exhaled through right absorption of oxygen and proper functioning of the lungs.

   • Regular pranayama, *nadi shodhana* (alternate nostril breathing), emphasizing the right nostril breath, heating forms of pranayama like *bhastrika* and *ujjayi* breathing.

   • Control of the motor organs, avoiding excess activity, particularly control of the speech and sexual organs.

3. Manasika Agni — Agni of the Mind

   • Balancing the mental agni: right balance of impressions taken in and expressions given out through proper absorption of impressions.

- Pratyahara practices including fasting from impressions and holding to uniform impressions.
- Visualization to control the senses from within.
- Subtle sensory tools of color, sound and music.
- Concentrating on the inner sounds and inner light.

4. Bauddhika Agni — Agni of the Intelligence

- Balancing the agni of intelligence: balanced judgment and reason through ability to discern between truth and falsehood.
- Study of spiritual teachings and philosophies.
- Cultivating right values and right judgments.
- Developing discrimination between the eternal and the transient.
- Equanimity and balanced judgment.
- Contemplation and meditation.

5. Anandagni — Agni of Bliss

- Balancing the Agni of experience: love, devotion and compassion.
- Right association and proper relationship.
- Worship of God, the Father/Mother and Creator of all.
- Respect for the guru, teachers and parents.
- Solitude (fasting from relationship).
- Steady remembrance of one's true nature.
- Samadhi and union with divine.

6. Chidagni — Agni of Consciousness

- Offering all experience in the fire of awareness.

- Observation, witnessing, silence of mind.
- Holding to the awareness of the immortal and immutable Self within the heart.
- Self-abidance and Self-realization.

7. Brahmagni — Divine Agni

- Seeing the unity of Being in all things.
- Offering all things to the One.
- Living in the Absolute.

9

Secrets of the Five Pranas

All that exists in the three heavens rests in the control
of Prana. As a mother her children, oh Prana,
protect us and give us splendor and wisdom.

PRASHNA UPANISHAD II.13

To change something we must alter the energy which creates it. This fact is true in the practice of yoga as well as in Ayurveda. To bring about positive changes in body and mind we must understand the energy through which they work. This is called *prana* in Sanskrit, meaning primary energy. It is sometimes translated as breath or vital force, though it is more than these.

While the subject of prana is common in yogic and ayurvedic thought, prana and its different subtypes are seldom examined in depth. For this reason, the vast and profound science of prana is rarely understood. In this chapter we will look into this force because prana is the main link between yoga and Ayurveda.

There is an old Vedic story about prana that occurs in various *Upanishads*. The five main faculties of our nature — the mind, breath (prana), speech, ear and eye — were arguing with each other as to which was the best and most important. This reflects the ordinary human condition in which our faculties are not integrated but fight with each other, competing for their rule over our attention. To resolve this dispute they decided that each would leave the body and see whose absence was most missed.

First speech left the body, but the body continued though mute. Next the eye left, but the body continued though blind. Next the ear left, but the body continued though deaf. Then the mind left, but the body continued though unconscious. Finally the prana began to leave and the body began to die and all the other faculties began to lose their energy. So they all rushed to prana and told it to stay, lauding its supremacy. Clearly prana won the argument. Prana gives energy to all our faculties, without which they cannot function. Prana takes the first place and without it we do not have the energy to do anything. The moral of this story is that to control all our faculties the key is the control of prana. Prana is the master. Prana is the boss. It is the power of God within us. Without the sanction of prana nothing can be done either at a voluntary or involuntary level in body and mind. Unless we learn how to work with our prana, we cannot get anything done.

Prana has many levels of meaning — from the breath to the energy of consciousness itself. Prana is not only the basic life-force, it is the master form of all energy working on the levels of mind, life and body. Indeed the entire universe is a manifestation of prana, which is the original creative power. Even kundalini shakti, the serpent power or inner force that transforms consciousness, develops from the awakened prana.

On a cosmic level there are two basic aspects of prana. The first is the unmanifest aspect of prana, which is the energy of pure consciousness that transcends all creation. The second or manifest prana is the force of creation itself. Prana arises from the quality (guna) of rajas, the active force of nature (Prakriti). Of the three gunas, sattva or harmony gives rise to the mind, rajas or movement gives rise to the prana, and tamas or inertia gives rise to the body.

Indeed it could be argued that Prakriti (nature) is primarily prana or rajas. Nature is an active energy or shakti. According to the pull or attraction of the higher Self or pure consciousness (Purusha), this energy becomes sattvic. By the inertia of ignorance this energy becomes tamasic.

However, the Purusha or higher Self can be said to be unmanifest prana because it is a form of energy of consciousness (*devatma shakti* or *citi shakti*). From the unmanifest prana of pure awareness comes the manifest prana of creation, through which the entire universe comes into being. From the unmanifest prana Purusha (energy of pure awareness), the prana Prakriti (energy of creation) manifests.

Relative to our physical existence, prana or vital energy is a modification of the air element, primarily the oxygen we breathe that allows us to live in the physical world. Yet as air originates in ether or space, prana arises in space and remains closely connected to it. Wherever we create space, there energy or prana must arise automatically. Air and space, energy and space, and energy and mind, which is a kind of space, remain closely linked and cannot be separated.

The element of air relates to the sense of touch, which is the subtle air element. Touch is the subtle form of prana. Through touch we feel alive and can transmit our life-force to others, which is why touch and embrace are so stimulating. Yet as air arises in space, so touch arises from sound, which is the sense quality that corresponds to the element of ether. Through sound we awaken and feel our broader connections with life as a whole. On a subtle level, prana arises from the touch and sound qualities that are inherent in the mind.

Pranamaya kosha is the sphere of our vital life energies. This sheath mediates between the body on one side and the three sheaths of the mind (outer mind, intelligence and inner mind) on the other and has an action on both levels. A good English term for the pranamaya kosha is the "vital sheath" or "vital body," a term from Sri Aurobindo's Integral Yoga. Pranamaya kosha consists of our vital urges of survival, reproduction, movement and self-expression, being mainly connected to the five motor organs (excretory, urinogenital, feet, hands, and vocal organ).

Most of us are dominated by the vital body and its deep-seated urges — such as eating and reproduction, which are animal in nature — that are necessary to sustain life. The vital body holds a vital or subconscious ego which is the source of the various fears, desires and attachments that cause us pain. Most of us spend our time in life seeking enjoyment through the vital body in the form of sensory pleasure and acquisition of material objects. The vital body, like prana, is dominated by the guna of rajas and its desires and passions.

A person with a strong vital nature becomes prominent in life and is able to impress his or her personality upon the world. Those with a weak vital nature lack the power to accomplish anything and have little effect upon life, usually remaining in subordinate positions. Generally, people with strong and egoistic vitals run the world, while those with weak vitals follow them. Such a strong egoistic vital is one of the greatest obstacles to the spiritual path. The person feels powerful in their ego identity and cannot surrender to any higher or impersonal force.

A strong vital or pranamaya kosha, however, is important for the spiritual path, but this is very different than the egoistic or desire-oriented vital. It derives its strength not from personal power but from surrender to the divine and the cosmic life force. Without a strong spiritual vital, we lack the power to do our practices. In Hindu mythology this higher prana is symbolized by the monkey-god Hanuman, the son of the Wind, who surrendered to the divine in the form of Sita-Rama. Hanuman can become as large or small as he wishes, can overcome all enemies and obstacles, and accomplish the miraculous. Such a spiritual vital has energy, curiosity and enthusiasm in life, along with a control of the senses and the subordination of the vital urges to a higher will and aspiration.

Health also depends upon a strong vital, which imparts energy and vigor to the physical body. But in Ayurveda true health is of the spiritualized vital nature, not of the egoistic vital. That is why ayurvedic health measures are based upon sattvic principles and attunement with the higher Self. Ayurveda aims at giving us health as attuned to the soul. Having a healthy ego, on the other hand, an ego with a lot of physical and vital strength, will only lead us into further karmic involvement and so harm our spiritual growth.

The Five Pranas

The one primary Prana divides into five types according to its movement and direction. These five pranas are called *vayus* or powers of air. They are an important subject in ayurvedic medicine and yogic thought, serving to link the two together. They represent the five types of energy that we have and through which all the universe operates.

Prana: literally the "forward moving air," moves inward. It governs reception of all types from the eating of food, drinking of water and inhalation of air to the reception of sensory impressions and mental experiences. Prana is propulsive in nature, setting things in motion and guiding them. It provides the basic energy that drives us in life. Prana is the vital energy in the head, primarily the region of the third eye, which nourishes the brain. It provides positive energy for all the other pranas.

Apana: literally the "air that moves away," moves downward and outward. It governs the elimination of the stool and the urine, the expelling of semen, menstrual fluid and the fetus, and the elimination of carbon dioxide through the breath. On a deeper level, apana rules the elimination of negative sensory, emotional and mental experiences. It is the basis of our immune function on all levels. Apana is the vital energy in the lower abdomen that allows for elimination and reproduction.

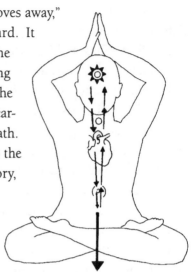

PRANA, APANA & UDANA

Udana: literally the "upward moving air," moves upward — the qualitative or transformative movements of the life-energy. It governs growth of the body, the ability to stand, speech, effort, enthusiasm and will. Udana is our main positive energy unfoldment in life through which we can develop our different bodies and evolve in consciousness. Udana is the vital energy in the throat that governs speech and self-expression and holds the head up through the neck.

Samana: literally the "balancing air," moves from the periphery to the center through a churning and discerning action. It aids in digestion on all levels. Samana works in the gastrointestinal tract to digest food, in the lungs to digest air or absorb oxygen, and in the mind to homogenize and digest experiences, whether sensory, emotional or mental. Samana is the vital energy in the navel, where our energy is centered and where digestion occurs.

Vyana: literally the "outward moving air," moves from the center to the periphery. It governs circulation on all levels. Vyana moves the food, water and oxygen throughout the body and keeps our emo-

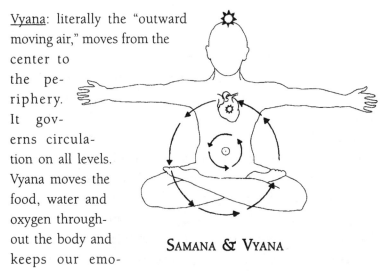

SAMANA & VYANA

tions and thoughts circulating in the mind, imparting movement and providing strength. In doing so it assists all the other pranas in their work. Vyana is the vital energy in the heart and lungs, where our energy expands.

While the action of the pranas can be localized to some degree, we must remember that it occurs on all levels because the main role of prana is to link things together. This is also why prana is not listed separately among the twenty-four cosmic principles of Samkhya. It is common to them all. Yet the pranas do govern different types of movement.

In terms of the physical body, prana vayu governs the movement of energy from the head down to the navel, which is the pranic center in the body. Apana vayu governs the movement of energy from the navel down to the root chakra and all the way down to the feet. Samana vayu governs the movement of energy from the entire body back to the navel. Vyana vayu governs the movement of energy out from the navel throughout the entire body. Udana governs the movement of energy from the navel up to the head. The navel is the main prana center in the body, in which all the pranas are held like the spokes in the center of a wheel.

As a simple summary, prana governs the intake of substances; samana governs their digestion; vyana governs the circulation of nutrients; udana governs the release of positive energy that follows digestion; and apana governs the elimination of waste materials. This is much like the working of a machine. Prana brings in the fuel. Samana converts the fuel into energy. Vyana circulates the energy to the various work sites. Apana releases the waste materials or by-products of the conversion process. Udana governs the positive energy created in the process and determines the work that the machine is able to do.

As a diagram of forces, samana governs the center while vyana governs the periphery. Udana governs upward movement, while apana governs downward movement. Prana gives energy to all the pranas. The key to health and well-being is to keep our pranas in harmony. When one prana becomes imbalanced, the others become disturbed as well because they are all linked together. Generally prana and udana work opposite to apana as the forces of energization versus those of elimination. Similarly vyana and samana are opposite as forces of expansion and contraction.

The pranas as forms of energy work on all the elements. Prana energizes the elements in whatever they do. Udana governs the upward transformation of the elements, allowing earth to become water, water to become fire, fire to become air and air to become ether. Apana governs the downward transformation, allowing ether to become air, air to become fire, fire to become water, and water to become earth. Vyana allows for the differentiation of the elements and grants each their separate sphere of activity. Samana brings about the integration of the elements and keeps them connected.

The pranas have specific elemental connections as well (though not everyone agrees on the specifics of these, even in classical yogic literature). Udana relates to ether and sound, which relate to the throat chakra. Vyana relates to air and touch, which relate to the heart chakra. Samana relates to fire and sight, which relate to the navel chakra. Apana relates to earth and water and to smell and taste, which relate to the root and sex chakras. Prana is connected to all the elements but more specifically to the water form of apana, which is the basis of life and procreation. Prana also rules the mind from its center in the head. Prana governs all forms of energy in the universe, not just that of the life-force but also material energies. Apana, for example, is connected to gravity. Light moves by the power of prana.

Prana prevails in the eastern direction which is the direction of light and life. Vyana prevails in the south, the direction of growth and expansion. Apana prevails in the west, the direction of decay and decline. Udana prevails in the north, the direction of death and ascension. Samana connects all the pranas together through space.

Prana also governs time. Prana propels the movement of time, which is the movement of life experience. It brings us into birth and carries us along our life journey. Vyana allows us to expand within the field of time. Apana causes us to decline. Udana allows us to move on in time to a higher sphere. Samana connects all the pranas through time.[22]

Prana	Stage of Life	Time of Day	Season	Direction
Prana	Birth	Sunrise	Spring	East - Above
Vyana	Growth	Noon	Summer	South - Front/Right
Apana	Decay	Sunset	Fall	West - Below
Udana	Death	Midnight	Winter	North - Back/Left
Samana	Life	Day	Year	Center

How Prana Creates the Physical Body

Without prana the physical body is no more than a lump of clay. Prana sculpts this gelatinous mass into various limbs and organs. It does this by creating various channels or nadis through which it can operate and energize gross matter into various tissues and organs.

Prana vayu creates the openings and channels in the head and brain. There are seven openings in the head: the two eyes, two ears, two nostrils and mouth. These are called the seven pranas or seven *rishis* in Vedic thought.[23] Udana creates the channels in the throat and neck, particularly those of the tongue and vocal organs. Both prana and udana help create the mouth which is the main opening in the head and in the body. It could be said that the entire physical body is an extension of the mouth — the main organ of physical activity, eating and self-expression.

Apana vayu creates the openings in the lower part of the body, those of the urinogenital and excretory systems. Samana vayu creates the openings in the middle part of the body, those of the digestive system, centered in the navel. It opens out into the channels of the intestines and the organs, like the liver and pancreas, which secrete into it. Vyana vayu creates the channels going to the peripheral parts of the body, the arms and legs. It creates the veins and arteries and also the muscles, sinews, joints and bones. Apana aids vyana in creating the legs, while udana supports it in creating the arms.

In summary, samana vayu creates the trunk of the body (which is dominated by the gastrointestinal tract), while vyana vayu creates the limbs. Prana and udana create the upper openings or bodily orifices, mainly the head, while apana creates those openings below in the lower abdomen.

Prana governs the upper part of the body (the head). Apana governs the lower part of the body. Vyana governs the front side of the body which connects to the limbs that mainly move forward. Udana governs the back, which allows the body to stand up. Samana connects all the parts of the body together in the navel.

In addition each prana relates to one of the seven bodily tissues. Prana creates the nerve tissue; apana creates the bone tissue; udana creates the muscle; samana creates the fat or adipose tissue; and vyana creates the connective tissue, sinews and ligaments (Sanskrit *snava*).[24]

Relative to the bodily organs, prana itself works mainly in the brain, senses and heart. Udana works in the stomach, lungs, and throat. Vyana works through the lungs and heart. Samana works through the digestive organs, particularly the small intestine, liver, stomach and pancreas. Apana works through the kidneys, urinary bladder and reproductive organs, the lower organs.

The Doshas, Tejas and Ojas

The five pranas are forms of vata, but all the doshas depend upon them for their right function both through expression and elimination. Udana vayu moves upward to eliminate kapha or mucus. This occurs through coughing, expectorating or vomiting, including the emetic therapy of pancha karma. Apana vayu moves downward to eliminate pitta (bile or toxic heat) through purgation, which is another method of pancha karma.

Samana increases agni, the digestive fire, which helps balance the doshas. This is the basis of the *shamana* or pacifying methodology of Ayurveda. Prana, by increasing intake of nutrients through the mouth and the senses, calms the doshas, particularly vata. This is part of tonification (*brimhana*) therapy. Vyana by outward motion promotes sweating and relieves toxins through the skin. This helps open the channels to draw the toxins back into the digestive tract for their elimination.

The five pranas have their connections with tejas and ojas as well. Apana governs ojas, which develops through the reproductive tissue. Samana controls tejas as not only the digestive fire but all other fires in the body and mind.

Disease mainly begins at the level of prana in the head, with head colds. It moves to the region of udana with sore throat. Then it descends to the region of vyana with lung infections. Deeper-seated digestive and metabolic problems then occur as pathogens move into the region of samana in the small intestine and liver. Finally toxins enter the region of apana in the kidneys and reproductive organs where they create long-term debility.

DEEPER LEVELS OF PRANA

Prana and the Breath

Prana exists on the level of pranamaya kosha, which is its native sphere. This impacts the physical body primarily through the breathing process, which is the main form of pranic activity in the body. In this regard prana governs inhalation. Samana governs absorption of oxygen that occurs mainly during retention of the breath. Vyana governs its circulation. Apana governs exhalation and the release of carbon dioxide. Udana governs the release of positive energy through the breath, including speech that occurs through the outgoing breath. We will discuss this more in the chapter on pranayama.

Prana and the Mind

The mind also has its energy or prana. This derives mainly from our intake of sensory impressions and is reflected in our expressions through our limbs and our speech.

Prana on a psychological level governs our receptivity to mental sources of nourishment, sensations, emotions and ideas. It gives energy, vitality and speed to the mind. When deranged, prana causes wrong desire and insatiable craving. We become misguided, misdirected and wrongly motivated. We run after things in the external world rather than following our own internal inspiration.

Apana on a psychological level governs our ability to eliminate negative thoughts and emotions, which become toxins in the mind. It gives us detachment and dispassion, functioning as our mental immune function. When deranged, apana causes fear and depression. We get clogged up with undigested experience that weighs us down in life, making us suppressed, stifled and weak.

Samana facilitates mental digestion, providing nourishment and contentment to the mind. It gives us mental discrimination, concentration and balance. Through it we can unite with what we put our minds and hearts upon. When deranged, samana brings about attachment and greed. We become contracted and tied up inside ourselves, clinging to wrong attitudes, beliefs and emotions.

Vyana promotes mental circulation, the free flow of ideas and emotions. It gives comprehensiveness, agility and independence to the mind. When deranged, vyana causes separation, hatred, and alienation. We are unable to unite with others or remain connected in what we do. We overly expand our energies to the point at which they dissipate or disintegrate.

Udana provides positive mental energy, will, and strength. It gives us joy and enthusiasm and helps awaken our higher spiritual and creative potentials. When deranged, udana causes pride, willfulness and arrogance. We become ungrounded, trying to rise too high, and lose track of our roots.

Prana therefore is our positive propulsive energy in life, our ability to move and develop. Apana is our capacity to withdraw our energy and to eliminate things from ourselves. Vyana is our capacity for self-expansion, while samana is our ability to hold and contract. Udana is our ability to ascend, rise up and grow. The five pranas are just the five expressions of our energy. Learning to use them, we can gain control over all aspects of our lives.

Spiritual Aspects of the Pranas

The pranas have many special actions in yogic practices. On a spiritual level, samana vayu governs the space within the heart in which the true Self, the Atman, dwells as a fire with seven flames. This is also called the internal space or atmosphere, *antariksha*, the hidden space between things. Samana regulates agni with fuel, which must burn evenly. Without the peace and balance of samana, we cannot return to the core of our being or concentrate the mind. Samana creates one-pointedness of mind that leads to samadhi.

Vyana governs the movement of prana through the nadis, keeping them open, clear, clean and even in their functioning. A strong vyana is necessary for purification of the nadis. It expands the mind into the infinite. Apana protects us from negative entities and experiences on the path. Prana itself gives us the proper aspiration and motivation for our spiritual development.

Udana governs our growth in consciousness and also brings about the movement up the sushumna. The mind moves with udana vayu.[25] This takes us to the states of dream and deep sleep. After death it leads the soul to the astral and causal planes. Udana is often the most important prana for spiritual growth.

As we practice yoga, the subtle aspects of these pranas begin to awaken. This may cause various unusual movements of energy in body and mind, including the occurrence of various spontaneous movements or *kriyas*. We may feel new expanses of energy (subtle vyana), great peace (subtle samana), a sense of lightness or levitation (subtle udana), deep groundedness and stability (subtle apana), or just heightened vitality and sensitivity (subtle prana).

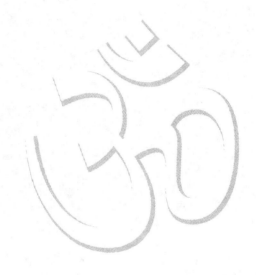

IO

Kundalini and the Chakras

Awakening the Subtle Body

Reverence to the Sushumna Nadi, to the Kundalini,
to the nectar born of the Moon, to the state in which
the mind is dissolved, reverence to the Goddess,
the Great Shakti, who is the Self of consciousness.

HATHA YOGA PRADIPIKA IV.64

The Seven Chakras

Yoga in the deeper sense requires awakening the kundalini or serpent power. Kundalini is the higher evolutionary force hidden within us that has the ability to unfold our spiritual potential. In its unawakened state, a mere fraction of its energy serves to uphold our normal psychophysical functioning. In its awakened state it reveals our capacity for cosmic consciousness, taking us beyond even what we could imagine.

These evolutionary potentials exist as latent energy centers in the subtle body, the seven chakras, which kundalini activates. *Chakra* refers to a wheel or a moving circle of energies. The chakras are also important in ayurvedic healing, particularly relative to the prana and mind, which works through them. The chakras direct and guide the physical body from behind the nervous system.

The seven chakras comprise three primary regions. The three

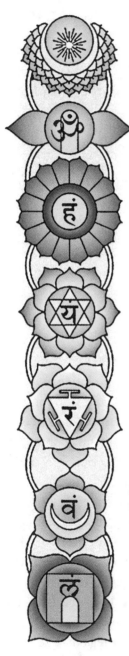

lower chakras are located close together from the base of the spine to the navel, a region of about six or eight inches. Together they are called the *kanda* or bulb and constitute the region of fire. The awakening kundalini lights up these three chakras together like a fire in a cauldron. The closeness of these chakras explains why in some texts the kundalini is said to rise from the root chakra, in others from the sex chakra, and yet others from the navel.

Similarly the three higher chakras — the throat, third eye and crown — are closely related and form the region of the head, governing the higher brain centers. They share many common qualities and powers of higher expression and perception. It is said to be the region of the moon, or *soma*, reflective and contemplative qualities.

In between stands the heart as the central chakra mediating between these two groups of three chakras, connecting both to the navel below and to the throat above. Sometimes the heart is included along with the three higher chakras. Other times it is placed along with the three lower. It is the region of the sun, which expands the light of fire and reflects its luminosity to the moon. It connects to the solar plexus between the heart and the navel.

THE CHAKRAS

The Threefold Head Chakra — Seat of the Moon

Sahasrara — Crown or Consciousness Chakra /the Moon
Ajna — Third Eye or Mind Chakra /Orb of the Moon
Visshuddha— Throat or Ether Chakra /Reflection of the Moon

The Central Heart — Seat of the Sun

Anahata — Heart or Air Chakra

The Threefold Kanda or Bulb — Seat of Fire

Manipura — Navel or Fire Chakra
Svadhishtana — Sex or Water Chakra
Muladhara — Root or Earth Chakra

The lower set of three chakras reflects more physical and vital functions, including most health issues, through the doshas. Vata has a special relationship with the root or earth chakra, which serves to stabilize it. Kapha connects with the water chakra. Pitta relates to fire. The heart chakra reflects emotional issues. The head chakras reflect spiritual issues. Similarly, there are three levels of working on the chakras relative to physical disease, psychological disease and spiritual growth.

1. Physical diseases relate to imbalances in outer chakra functioning through the various nerve plexus and endocrine organs with which the chakras correspond and to the three doshas of vata, pitta and kapha.

2. Psychological diseases involve imbalances in inner chakra functioning, particularly relative to prana, tejas and ojas, which are the energies of the subtle body, the mind and its field of impressions.

3. Spiritual or yogic development aims at opening the chakras.

This requires transcending their ordinary functions in our personal nature to the level of the cosmic. Yogis merge the chakras of the astral body into the causal body, reversing the entire process of creation. They merge earth into water, water into fire, fire into air, air into ether, ether into mind, mind into intelligence, and intelligence into the Supreme Self.

Most chakra healing today emphasizes external measures of gems, herbs, body work, sound, color therapy, and vibrational healing. In addition, psychic healers can work on the chakras through their own prana or chi, which they direct as a healing force. Ayurveda employs such modalities for treating disease and promoting health and vitality. These approaches are very important for chronic conditions, weak immunity, and deep-seated diseases of the nervous system.

Most books on chakras today describe the chakras as force centers within the physical body, with the *sushumna* or central channel identified with the spine. They relate the chakras to the various spinal centers and the physiological processes these govern like digestion, respiration or reproduction. Yet while the chakras do impact the physical body, which they form and energize, they are not themselves physical.

Some healers claim that working on the chakras with such outer methods can open or awaken the chakras. These statements must be taken with caution. According to yoga, in the ordinary human state, which it is extremely difficult to transcend except by sustained spiritual practice, the chakras remain closed; that is, they do not directly function at all. The result of this is not necessarily disease but spiritual ignorance. This consists of regarding the external world as the true reality and living unaware of one's true Self, which is neither body nor mind but thought-free awareness.

One's chakras can be closed on a spiritual level and yet one can be healthy, emotionally balanced, mentally creative, and successful in life. This depends upon outer, not inner chakra functioning. Opening the chakras is not a process for improving one's capacity in the regular domains of human life, though it may offer this as a sidelight, but for going beyond the ordinary human condition to a higher evolutionary state. The chakras can only be truly opened through inner practices of pranayama, mantra and meditation. Outer aids, from diet to gems, can be helpful but must remain subordinate to these higher modalities for optimal application.

Much of our thinking today, even in spiritual and New Age fields, is still cast in a materialistic paradigm in which we try to reduce everything to specific time-space coordinates. This mentality is used to approach subtle phenomena like the chakras, pranas or doshas. However, it is wrong to think that the chakras are like the limbs and organs of the physical body that can have little variability in their form, function or appearance. The chakras are energetic and functional centers, not physical positions. We experience them at certain points in the physical body more so than others but their action impacts the entire physical body, the mind and what is beyond as well. The result is that the chakras work in different ways at different times and for different people. They can be correlated with various phenomena on different levels relative to how the energy is working through them. For this reason all books on the chakras, including yogic accounts, may not agree in every detail. Such views may represent different insights or different methods of working with the chakras. They are not necessarily wrong, but traditional yoga teachings on the chakras should be given priority, given the long experiential tradition behind them.

The subtle body is the body of our impressions and our pranas. Can one put an impression in a box? Like the wind, prana has its movement, but it cannot be limited to a particular

TABLE OF CHAKRAS

Name	Muladhara	Svadhisthana	Manipura	Anahata	Visshuddha	Ajna	Sahasra Padma
Meaning	Root	Self-abode	City of Gems	Unstruck Sound	Very Pure	Command	Thousand Petalled Lotus
Location	Base/Earth	Sex/Water	Navel/Fire	Heart/Air	Throat/Ether	Third Eye	Top of head
Petals	4	6	10	12	16	2	1000
Bija Mantra	LAM	VAM	RAM	YAM	HAM	KSHAM	OM
Element	Earth	Water	Fire	Air	Ether	Mind Space	Consciousness Space
Symbol	Yellow Square	White Crescent Moon	Red Triangle	Gray Six Pointed Star	Azure Dot		
Animal	Elephant	Crocodile	Ram	Deer	Elephant		
Sense Organ	Nose	Tongue	Eye	Skin	Ears	Mind	Consciousness
Motor Organ	Excretory	Urino-Genital	Feet	Hands	Vocal Organ	Mind	Consciousness
Tanmatra	Smell	Taste	Sight	Touch	Sound	Thought	Consciousness
Color	Crimson Red	Vermilion	Dark Blue	Deep Red	Smoky Gray	Silver White	Colorless
Nadi	Alambusha	Kuhu	Vishvodhara	Varuna	Sarasvati	Ida, Pingala	Sushumna
Tissue	Muscle	Fat	Blood	Plasma	Prana	Subtle Prana	Causal Prana
Dosha	Kapha	Kapha	Pitta	Vata	Vata		
Prana	Apana	Apana	Samana	Vyana	Udana		

organ. Can one say where the wind is located or where it goes when it ceases to blow? Correlations are means of drawing connections and, as connections are ultimately universal in the spiritual realm, such correlations must have variability. We must learn to look at the subtle body according to its own reality that encompasses and interpenetrates physical reality on many levels, not which is simply parallel to physical functioning. The subtle body creates its own time and space, like a dream or a vision. It is not limited by external factors and forms.

Moreover, the opened chakras are not part of the ordinary functioning of the astral body either. They relate to its heightened or spiritually awakened role. They represent the absorption of the astral body back into the causal body and pure consciousness beyond. As the chakras are opened, the astral body is gradually dissolved. While we can correlate physical and subtle body components and functions, we should realize that the two are not the same, and the spiritually opened astral body is yet something more, resembling more a mist of energies spreading beyond the galaxies than something we can define in bodily terms.

Kundalini and the Chakras

The chakras are part of a much higher energy system than the physical body. To make a helpful analogy: activating each chakra requires doubling the amount of energy required for sustaining all ordinary body and brain functions. It requires about twice the energy to activate the first, the root or earth chakra, than the energy required for sustaining our ordinary psychophysical functions, twice that amount to activate the next chakra, and so on up to the top of the head. So there is a greater change of consciousness between chakras than from the ordinary human consciousness to the first awakened chakra.

For the chakras to come into function depends upon a higher source of energy than the physical body can provide. This is the role of the kundalini shakti. Kundalini is not a physical force, nor something that the ordinary mind or ego can control. It is the concentrated energy of awareness or attention. Only if a person has one-pointedness of mind can kundalini come into function in an harmonious manner. Kundalini is not an energy apart from consciousness, but the energy of awareness that manifests when the mind becomes free from the fragmentation of thought and emotion based on the ego.

The awakening of kundalini requires that the prana or life-force enters into the sushumna or central channel. This occurs when the prana is withdrawn from its fixation on the external world and removed from our sensory involvement. As long as our life-energy is identified with the physical body and its functions, it cannot come into the central channel. For this reason, the arousing of the kundalini involves a state of samadhi in which we leave ordinary consciousness. In the beginning this is experienced in a condition of trance in which we become unconscious of the physical body. Later it can occur in the waking state, without an impairment of physical action, but the physical body is no longer experienced as one's true identity.

Developing the awakened prana or kundalini energy greatly enhances one's skill and power as a healer. Kundalini is the very healing power of the Divine Mother that connects with cosmic life and love and its curative power. Such a healer can heal by mere touch, by their voice or by their presence. For this reason we should be careful not to try to manipulate this subtle pranic force but let the divine direct it for us. It is best to meditate upon the Divine Mother as wielding the pranic healing force, not ourselves personally. Power is always a temptation for the ego and, as kundalini is perhaps the greatest power, the ego may wish to catch it. But it is like seeking to catch lightning. One may only end up struck down.

Cosmic Aspects of Chakras

The opened chakras afford access to the cosmic functions of their respective elements and faculties. They give knowledge of the unity of the objective constituents of the universe (elements), the instruments of cognition (sense organs), and the instruments of action (organs of action), which are the subjective constituents of the universe. When the chakras are opened we experience the cosmic nature of these factors as part of our own deeper awareness. We learn the secrets of creation and merge the universe into our own minds.[26]

As we awaken our subtle energies and faculties, we may experience subtle sounds, lights, or visions of deities in the region of the third eye. But such experiences may come long before any particular chakra is opened. To bring the subtle centers into function, the gross or physical centers must be put in state of rest or equilibrium. That is why the practices of yoga develop stillness of body, breath, senses and mind, particularly through pratyahara as the basis for working with the chakras. Kundalini is a force of withdrawal, reversing the process of creation so that we can return to the One. Therefore it cannot function unless we reduce external involvement and attachments.

To properly develop the earth chakra requires detachment from the earth element. One no longer seeks to accumulate matter outwardly but learns to appreciate it inwardly as a form of perception. One learns to enjoy the colors, textures, and shadows of the earth element like a display of magnificent mountains within the mind, but one has no desire to possess or hold them.

To properly open the water chakra is different than having a heightened sexual drive or even great sexual potency. It requires that the physical sexual organ goes into a state of latency and the sexual drive is sublimated into a force of awareness. One learns to enjoy the flow and flavor of the water element as a movement of delight, riding on the waves of perception in the cosmic sea.

To properly open the fire chakra does not involve increasing one's personal will or determination. It requires awakening the cosmic energy of fire (tejas) and letting it blaze forth. One must oneself become a fire and burn all the impurities within the body and mind. It is like experiencing the fire that destroys the universe at the end of the cycle of the *yugas*, in which our personal motivations are effaced.

To open the heart or air chakra is quite different than to be in a heightened, vulnerable or open emotional state. To awaken the heart chakra we must go beyond personal emotions and understand the cosmic energy of love behind all emotional fluctuations. This requires an opening to the universal feelings of compassion and devotion, and contact with the universal life-force. It is an experience of pure devotion, becoming love itself.

To open the throat or ether chakra is not a matter of heightened speech or expression but of being silent in the expanse of cosmic space, in which our personal voice is lost in the divine Word. It is merging into the cosmic ether in which the essence of sound abides as eternal knowledge.

Opening the third eye requires learning to live as pure insight, not requiring a body or even senses. Opening the crown chakra means becoming one with the infinite, eternal nature of pure Existence in which separate self disappears.

The awakening of the consciousness behind the subtle body involves being able to take off the gross body and its functions like a heavy overcoat which is no longer necessary on a warm summer day. This can be frightening to those attached to the body, but it is delightful to those who do not perceive life in limited terms.

Chakras, Experiences and Powers

Each chakra provides an awareness of corresponding levels of the universe or different worlds (lokas) beyond the physical. We gain insights into the subtle workings of nature (Prakriti), the senses and their subtle essences (tanmatras), the life-force (pranas), and the process of cosmic creation.

The corresponding subplanes of the astral universe, which are quite marvelous beyond anything in the physical world, may become available to the third eye. Beautiful astral mountains may be seen, vast expanses of translucent astral oceans, scintillating astral suns and pulsating astral stars. One may ride the astral winds through various worlds, or expand one's mind through endless astral spaces and their many universes of beauty and delight. One can meet with sages and deities or with friends from former lives, renewing soul connections. In the higher chakras one can gain access to causal realms of pure insight, ideal perception, and endless awareness beyond personal limitation. One can visit the workshop of creation and see how the universes are made out of mind and thought alone.

Yet not all yogis choose to explore the worlds or the faculties that relate to the chakras. Many great *jnanis*, or yogis of the path of knowledge, strive to merge directly into pure unity or the Absolute, which is beyond both subtle and causal bodies. In their awakening they may hardly note the distinctions of the chakras and their functions. From their experience — such as that of Ramana Maharshi, who perhaps most typifies this view — there is only one chakra or center which is that of the Self in the heart, from which all the phenomenon of the gross and subtle worlds and bodies appear like images seen in a mirror or bubbles on the waves of the sea. Similarly many great devotees simply seek to merge in God or *Bhagavan* in the heart and are not concerned with the various experiences of the chakras, even when these are known to them. These are very high states that few can approach, but we must recognize that the chakras are a series of stages rather than an end in themselves, and can become a side track if we are not careful.

Yogic literature speaks of various *siddhis* or psychic powers. These relate primarily to the subtle body and its pranas, as subtle matter is totally malleable. The subtle udana or upward-moving air allows one to become as light as one likes, including the ability to levitate (*laghima*). The subtle apana or downward-moving air enables us to become as heavy or as stable as we wish (*garima*). The subtle vyana or expansive air allows us to become as large as we like, to expand endlessly (*mahima*). The subtle samana or contracting air allows us to become as small as we like, to be perfectly concentrated (*anima*). The primary prana itself allows us to gain whatever we wish (*prapti*). As the chakras open, these corresponding powers in the subtle body may be experienced. Sometimes their effects extend into the physical body as well.

In addition we should not forget that many subtle states exist between ordinary physical consciousness and the true awakening of the kundalini and the chakras. We should not regard any extraordinary experience as enlightenment or as a kundalini experience. Visions, out-of-body experiences, trances, channeling, mystical dreams, genius, inspiration of various sorts and other such states, even if legitimate, may still fall short of the real awakening of the kundalini and certainly should not be confused with Self-realization, which requires the full development of our awareness rather than giving ourselves over to some entity or experience outside ourselves.

To properly open the chakras requires divine grace. It cannot be done willfully or forcefully arrived at from a state of emotional disturbance. Attempts to awaken kundalini without having first purified the body and mind lead to side effects in which the mind or the life-force become disturbed and various illusory experiences arise. For this reason, traditional yogic literature has always stressed right living factors and right attitudes (yamas and niyamas), as well as appropriate ayurvedic lifestyle regimens, as the basis for kundalini practices.

While it is possible to have aberrant kundalini or chakra experiences, most of these are pranic or mental disturbances. If the mind is not purified there can be a heightened activity of the lower chakras, along with an increase in their corresponding physical and emotional urges. For this reason we should seek to work on the lower chakras from the standpoint of the higher, mainly either the heart or the third eye.

In addition to the seven higher chakras, there are seven lower chakras beneath the muladhara which relate to the underworld, the lower astral or realm of the *asuras* (anti-Gods), the powers that work to keep us in ignorance and illusion. It is possible to fall into these lower chakras and their negative experiences of wrath, pride and power if one is not careful.

If we approach the chakras carefully and with the right guidance, we have nothing to fear, but it is better to be overly cautious rather than too daring while working with these lightning-like forces. Above all we should understand that opening the chakras is not an end itself, but part of the process of Self-realization. The chakras only show the road; they also indicate the side paths where one can go astray. While we need to understand them, we must do so in terms of their cosmic connections.

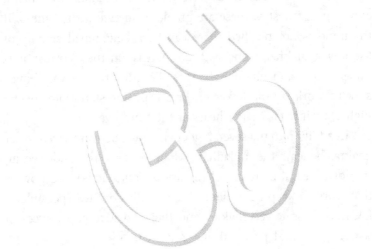

II

The Nadis

The Channel Systems of Mind and Prana

*When all the knots of the heart are broken,
then the mortal becomes immortal.*

KATHA UPANISHAD 6.15

Ayurveda views the body as a collection of channels from the great channel that is the gastrointestinal tract to the subtle channels of the nervous system. Yoga similarly looks upon the subtle body (mind-prana field) as a system of interrelated channels (nadis). The channels in the physical body interconnect with the channels of the subtle body.

According to the Vedic view, Vayu, the cosmic air force, creates all these channels. Vayu is called *sutratman*, the Self or Atman of the sutra, meaning a thread, channel or canal. The channels created by Vayu hold all things in the universe like gems on a string. Just as there are channels in the body, so external nature is filled with various channels — from rivers and streams to currents of energy in intergalactic space. In this section we will discuss the channels of the mind and the subtle body. General books on Ayurveda can be consulted for information on the physical channels.

Chitta Nadi, the Mind or Consciousness Channel

The mind has its own single nadi or channel called *chitta nadi* or the channel of consciousness. Ayurveda refers to its physical counterpart as *manovaha strotas*, the channel that carries thought. All of us have experienced the flow of the mind, the flow of thought or the stream of consciousness. This is the flow through the chitta nadi.

Chitta nadi originates in the spiritual heart, the site of the reincarnating soul or individual Self, Jivatman. In the heart resides our connection with the Creator from which the chitta nadi gains energy. The core impulses arising from our deeper mind or heart, our samskaras, propel the movement through this nadi.

Chitta nadi is the flow of our samskaras from the heart to the outer world. It moves upward first to the throat, from which our expression comes out, and then to the head where it gets connected with the senses and external objects. Then it flows back down from the head to the throat and back to the heart. This is the twofold flow of the chitta nadi. First it has a movement out toward the external world, which is from the heart up to the head and out through the senses. Then it has a contrary movement from the outer world of the senses to the inner world of the psyche, which is down from the head into the heart.

The outward flow of the chitta nadi gives rise to the outer mind, emotions, and life urges, what Samkhya calls the field of manas and the subtle body. The inner flow of the chitta nadi gives rise to the inner mind and intuition, what Samkhya calls buddhi or inner intelligence.[27] The outward flow follows the movement of the cosmic repulsive force or ignorance. The inward flow reflects the movement of divine attraction. The outward flow of chitta nadi brings us into the body and creates the waking state, which is dominated by sensory activity in the head. The inner flow of the chitta nadi takes us into our own consciousness and creates the states of dream and deep sleep. Dream occurs in the throat region. Deep sleep occurs at the origin of the heart.

THE TWOFOLD FLOW OF THE MIND CHANNEL

	Head	
	Ego-identity, Ahamkara I am the body idea	
	Diversified Prana	
Outward Flow		Inward Flow
Manas,		Buddhi, Inner
Outer Mind		Intelligence
Sensation		Knowledge
	Heart, Chitta	
	Self or Soul (Jivatman) Core Mind, Samskaric Field	
	Original Prana	

At death, the chitta nadi flows inward, as in sleep, taking us into the astral plane and its dream-like experience of heaven and hell worlds. The tunnel experiences that people commonly have in near-death experience show the functioning of this nadi.

In the ordinary human mind, the flow through the chitta nadi is restricted and broken up. Our minds are distracted and fragmented and move in various directions. Nevertheless there remains some consistency to the flow through the mind channel, which we experience as our self-identity. The dominant thought flowing through chitta nadi is the I-thought. The identification of the self with the body generates the external flow of chitta nadi. The recognition of the Self as pure consciousness generates the internal flow.

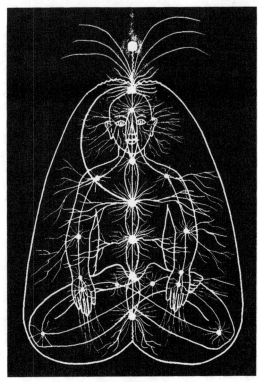

THE NADIS

Ego (*ahamkara*) is the factor that brings about the restriction of flow through the chitta nadi. It is the negative movement of prana in the mind, while the soul or sense of divine Self is the positive movement of prana in the mind. Ego is a manifestation of deranged or desire-based prana (apana in the mind), while the soul reflects balanced or love-based prana.

When the chitta nadi is blocked by the thought of the separate self, we get trapped in the outer mind, emotions and senses. As we expand our sense of self from the personal to the universal, the flow in chitta nadi increases. When the chitta nadi flows freely it completes its circuit and returns to the heart. In the practice of meditation one can experience this quicker, freer and more consistent flow through chitta nadi. Once the flow becomes completely liberated, it merges us back into the ocean of consciousness that dwells within the heart; the free flow becomes one with silence and stillness.

Ego causes various toxins, impurities or heavy matters (*malas*) to accumulate in the chitta nadi and inhibit its flow. These toxins derive from wrongly digested food, impressions and associations, from wrong diet, wrong use of the senses, and wrong relationships. Hence the flow through the chitta nadi is affected by the condition of the body, prana and mind. Chitta nadi is connected to all the channel systems of the physical and subtle bodies.

In this regard, yoga speaks of the knots in the heart (*hridaya granthi*) that must be untied for liberation or enlightenment to occur. These knots are the constrictions in the flow of the chitta, blockages in the flow of vayu or prana in the mind space. Our samskaras, deep desires or impulses inhibit the flow of energy from the Self through the chitta nadi and get projected into the external world as various limited ego identities. Opening the spiritual heart and opening the chitta nadi are thus the same. Along with the chitta nadi, related peripheral subtle nadis open, bringing an experience of bliss into the physical body itself.

In fact the mind is not different from its flow. The vibration of the mind (*chitta-spanda*) is the flow of the mind (chitta nadi). When the mind comes to a state of calm and silence, then the flow of the mind channel also becomes calm, merging into peace, expanding into space.

Chitta Nadi and the Other Channels

Chitta nadi is the channel of the causal body, the field of the deeper mind and heart. From it arises the original prana of the soul that is the basis of all life. Chitta nadi, therefore, is the original pranic flow as well as that of the mind. The movement of the mind (chitta-spanda) is always reflected in the movement of prana (prana-spanda). As such, chitta nadi governs over all channel functioning. It is most intimately related to the sushumna, the governing channel of the subtle body, and to the kundalini, the serpent power which is the awakened flow of energy through the sushumna. The free flow through the chitta nadi causes the kundalini to flow through the sushumna as well. Chitta nadi relates to the upper regions of the sushumna from the heart to the head.

Chitta nadi governs not only the flow of thought but also the flow of prana that derives from it. The sushumna as the higher pranic nadi is closely connected with the chitta nadi or channel of the mind in its awakened flow. When the chitta nadi flows outward, the kundalini remains asleep or dormant. When chitta nadi flows within, then kundalini awakens and begins to move.

The inward flow of the chitta nadi leads to the purification and energization of all the other nadis, leading to the opening of the chakras and their potentials. However, not all yogis will experience all the chakras and their energies. Some may go directly to the heart and not concern themselves with the other possibilities of experience.

The flow of chitta nadi is desire based. Desire causes the chitta nadi to flow outward. Detachment allows it to flow within. As sexual desire is the strongest desire, it has the greatest outward pull on this channel. As the chitta nadi flows outward, our energy gets directed to the external world, where it is eventually lost. As it flows within, our energy gets directed within for internal transformation.

In terms of yogic practices, pratyahara (control of the senses) works to inhibit the outward flow through chitta nadi so that the inward flow can be developed. Dharana is the concentration of energy in the chitta nadi through directed attention. Meditation occurs when the energy flows continuously through chitta nadi. Samadhi occurs when the chitta nadi flows without obstruction. Perhaps the best method is to follow the current of thought back to its origin in the I-thought in the heart, the divine "I-am-that-I-am" which is the essence of the yoga of knowledge. Another way is to worship God in the heart in whatever form appeals to us. Mantra or anything else that creates a constant stream of higher thoughts helps open chitta nadi.

Anything that expands our consciousness will similarly cause its energy to flow more freely. In other words, all of yoga, particularly its higher practices, aims at developing the chitta nadi. Among the doshas, the chitta nadi is most closely related to vata, owing to vata's connection with prana and with the mind. Mind, prana and vata move together. Vata aggravation brings about abnormal or disturbed flow through the chitta nadi. However, kapha as attachment can block its flow. Pitta as anger similarly can agitate its flow. Relative to the three vital essences, prana arises through the free flow of chitta nadi. Tejas is its light power. Ojas is the stability of its flow.

The Fourteen Channels of the Subtle Body

The subtle body contains seventy-two thousand nadis. The most important fourteen of these rule over all mind-body functions. Of them, three determine the primary energy flows and one holds the key to spiritual development.

The Sushumna

The most important and central of these nadis is called the sushumna or astral spine. It is located in the spinal canal in the physical body. It controls all the functions of various chakras that are placed like lotuses upon it. The sushumna is sattvic in nature and becomes activated by the awakened kundalini or prana shakti. Otherwise its energy flow is very limited.

Ida and Pingala

The *ida* and *pingala* along with the sushumna are the three most important nadis. When the sushumna is not awakened, the energy flows through one of these two channels alternately, which complement each other in their work. They run to the left and right of the sushumna like two interwoven spirals from its origin at the base of the spine to the region of the third eye, ending at the left and the right nostrils.

The ida is the left nadi. It has a lunar, feminine, cooling or kapha energy and is tamasic in quality. Ida provides inspiration of vision, speech and imagination and elevates our devotional inclinations, making us more caring and loving. The pingala is the right nadi. It has a solar, masculine, heating or pitta energy and is rajasic in quality. Pingala provides motivation, drive, and determination and allows us to pursue deeper knowledge and perception.

Normally our energy flows more in one nadi than the other, which we can determine by examining the nostril through which the breath is mainly flowing. In this regard the two nadis relate to right and left brain functioning. Left brain functioning relates to the opposite or right nadi and makes us rational, independent and aggressive. Right brain functioning relates to the opposite or left nadi and makes us emotional, sensitive and receptive. When the breath is more in the left nostril, the right brain and its functions get activated. When it is more on the right side, the left brain and its functions are promoted.

When the prana or life-force is balanced, when the energy in the solar and lunar nadis is equalized, then the kundalini awakens and the prana enters the sushumna. This brings the subtle body into function and takes us into a higher state of mind and perception. The key to health of the subtle body lies in balancing the flow of energy through these two nadis. Note the chapter on pranayama for more information in this regard.

If we try to awaken the kundalini or open the chakras while the nadis are not balanced, we can drive subtle toxic substances into the sushumna or into the ida and pingala. The kundalini moving into the ida will cause false imaginations and distorted emotions, an overly passive mind, along with a possible loss of consciousness to other entities. Generally, kapha disorders and overweight will occur on a physical level. Moving into the pingala, the kundalini will cause anger, self-righteousness and an overly critical mind, an egoistic person who thinks that they are very spiritual. On a physical level, fever, inflammation and internal heat of a mysterious origin will develop.

The Fourteen Major Nadis

Along with the three main nadis, eleven more are important, making fourteen major nadis. Each nadi is identified by the point (aperture) in the body that it is connected to. All nadis begin at the root chakra or base of spine, follow the course of the sushumna and branch out at certain points along the spine. Eight nadis follow the right/left predominance of the ida and pingala. Six relate to the six chakras.

Nadis on the Right Side (Pingala Predominant)

1. Pingala: "The Red" — branches out from the third eye, goes to the right nostril, which its orifice, and supplies prana to it; also governs the right nasal passage.

2. Pusha: "The Nourisher" — a form of the Sun God, branches out from the third eye, goes to the right eye, which is its orifice, and supplies prana to it. It is mainly ruled by prana. This is a very important nadi because the soul (Atman) dwells in the right eye during the waking state. Meditation upon the Seer in the right eye is a major approach to Self-realization.

3. Payasvini: "Full of Juice" — branches out from the third eye, goes to the right ear, which is its orifice, and supplies prana to it; it also governs the right Eustachian tube. At the right ear we hear the inner sounds or nada.

4. Yashasvati: "Abounding in Glory" — runs from root chakra

to the navel chakra where it branches out. Supplies prana to the right foot and right hand. Its energy comes to a center in the middle of the hand and foot and from there radiates out to the five fingers or toes, ending primarily in the thumb and big toe. Its apertures are the tip of the thumb and the big toe. There is a strong healing energy possible through the palm of the right hand, which like the right eye often relates to the soul.

Nadis on the Left Side (Ida Predominant)

1. Ida: "The Inspirer" — branches out from the third eye, goes to the left nostril, which is its orifice, and supplies prana to it; it also governs the left nasal passage. It also governs inspired or visionary speech. It causes the whole body to be nourished through prana.

2. Shankhini: "Like a Sea Shell" — branches out from the third eye, goes to the left ear, which is its orifice, and supplies prana to it; also governs the left Eustachian tube. It makes us receptive to higher influences.

3. Gandhari: A musical note — Branches out from the third eye. It goes to the left eye, which is its orifice, and supplies prana to it. Also promotes dream and creative vision.

4. Hastijihva: "The Elephant's Tongue" — runs from the root chakra to the navel chakra where it branches out. Supplies prana to the left foot and left hand. Its energy comes to a center in the middle of the hand and foot and from there radiates out to the five fingers or toes, ending primarily in the thumb and big toe. Its apertures are the tip of the thumb and big toe.

Central Nadis

1. Alambusha: Refers to a barrier or a limit — runs from the

base of the spine or center of the root chakra back to the tip of the rectum and supplies prana to the organs of elimination. Its aperture is the anus. It relates to the root or earth chakra and is connected to apana.

2. Kuhu: "The Hidden or New Moon" — runs from the base of the spine to the sex chakra and forward to the end of the penis or vagina, supplying prana to the reproductive organs as well as to the urinary organs connected to them. Its aperture is the penis or vagina. It relates to the sex or water chakra and is connected to apana.

3. Vishvodhara: "The Carrier of All" — runs from the base of the spine to the navel chakra and to the stomach; it supplies prana to the digestive system. Its aperture is the navel. It relates to the navel or fire chakra and is connected to samana.

4. Varuna: "The Pervader" — a Vedic god who governs the cosmic Ocean of Space. It runs from the base of the spine to the heart chakra and supplies prana to the entire body, generally through the respiratory, circulatory and sebaceous systems. Its aperture is the skin. It relates to the heart or air chakra and to vyana. This nadi allows for the deeper feeling and knowing of the heart to manifest.

5. Sarasvati: "The Goddess of Speech" — branches out from the throat chakra. It goes to the tip of the tongue and supplies prana to it. It also covers the mouth and throat generally. It relates to the throat or ether chakra and to udana. This nadi, as the name indicates, gives the powers of speech, wisdom and mantra.

6. Sushumna : "The Very Blissful" — goes from the base of the spine or center of the root chakra to the top of the head. It also

energizes the spine, the brain, the nerve tissue and supports the bone. In the region of the third eye it collects the energy of all the other nadis, particularly the eight right-left predominant nadis. It is connected to prana among the five pranas.

Placement of the Nadis

The body has seven orifices above in the head: the right and left nostrils, the right and left ears, the right and left eyes, and the mouth. These are called the seven rishis or sages because they are our guiding faculties. They are also called the seven pranas because they govern over different forms of prana and the seven suns (*Adityas*) because they allow for various forms of illumination. They are said to be gods or *devas* whose guru is *Brihaspati* (speech).

There are two orifices below, the urethra and anus. These are said to be the demons or asuras whose guru is *Shukra* (reproduction). Along with the navel, there are ten orifices. The point at the top of the head is the eleventh and is related to the mind or consciousness.

These cover eleven of the fourteen nadis. The foot and hand nadis have energy openings to the external world through the hands and feet. The skin itself is an opening for the entire body. These make up the remainder of the fourteen nadis.

All fourteen nadis end at different apertures of the body, which they supply. They arise from the base of the spine. Only two, the sushumna and the alambusha, arise directly from the center of the root chakra. The others arise from the small triangle around the center. Only in the case of spiritual awakening does the prana directly enter the sushumna. Otherwise it remains in the peripheral twelve nadis, dominated by ida and pingala and their left and right side predominance.

Our energy generally rises through the sushumna and

sarasvati. It is drained downwards by alambusha and kuhu. The pure prana rises through sushumna; the impure prana dissipates through alambusha.

As the pingala and ida move around each other from chakra to chakra in a spiral fashion, up to the right and left nostrils carrying the solar and lunar forces, so do payasvini and shankhini move to the right and left ear, pusha and gandhari to the right and left eye, while yashavati and hastijihva move to the right and left sides of the body. These eight channels are related and usually function together. When the prana is on the right side flowing through the pingala, it is also usually flowing in the right ear, right eye and right side of the body through the respective channels. When it is flowing through the ida, it is also in the left ear, left eye, and left side of the body.

The five senses have their respective channels: for hearing, those to the right and left ear (payasvini and shankhini); for touch, that to the skin (varuna); for sight, those to the right and left eye (pusha and gandhari); for taste, that to the tongue (sarasvati); for smell, those to the right and left nostril (pingala and ida). The five organs of action have their respective channels: for speech (sarasvati), for the hands and feet (yashasvati and hastijihva), for the urinogenital organs (kuhu) and for the anus (alambusha).

Treatment of the Fourteen Nadis

The best way to treat the nadis is to treat their different orifices or apertures, which are their main sites for reception and transmission of energy. This can be done through massage, heat therapy (like the burning of moxa) or the application of herbs and oils. Prana moves through the channels, coming in and out of the body, creating these different openings. By treating these channels we can influence all the pranas and energies of the body and mind.

The sushumna can be treated by applying pressure to the point at the top of the head, by massage of the scalp or the application of herbs and oils. Brahmi oil (gotu kola prepared in a coconut oil base) is specific for lubricating and tonifying the sushumna and head center.

The channels to the ear (payasvini and shankhini) can be stimulated by pressing the lobe of the ear or by massage of the ear. They can be tonified by oil massage to the opening of the ear. Brahmi oil also is very good for them.

The channels to the eyes (pusha and gandhari) can be stimulated by pressing the points around the eyes, particularly the point central and above the eyes. Oils and herbs applied to the eyes are also useful. Triphala ghee is best for this. The eyes can also be balanced or stimulated by applying pressure or oils to the third eye, particularly sandalwood paste or sandalwood oil.

The channels to the nose (pingala and ida) can be stimulated by pressing the points immediately to the right and left of the nostrils. They can also be treated by alternative nostril breathing and by *nasya* therapies (mainly with calamus), as well as by aromatherapy (spicy oils like camphor, mint or cinnamon). These two channels are, of course, the most important in treatment because we can deal with them directly through the breath.

The channels to the feet and hand (yashasvati and hastijihva) are perhaps the most important for treatment as well as the easiest to manipulate externally. Through them we can balance the pranic flows in the entire body. These two nadis relate to various small or secondary chakras or nadi centers that radiate out from them in the region of the joints (shoulder, elbow, wrist, and hand, hip, knee, ankle and foot). They can be treated by massage of the hands and feet, particularly the fingers and toes, as well as by massage of the limbs, particularly in the region of the joints. Applying pressure to the center of the foot or hand and to the ends of the fingers or toes is helpful. Herbs and oils can be applied to the palms of the hands and soles of the feet to work on them.

The channel to the tongue (sarasvati) can be treated by application of herbs and oils to the neck and throat. Calamus ghee is particularly good. Placing the tongue at the roof of the mouth is helpful in connecting the sarasvati with the sushumna.

The whole body channel (varuna) can be treated by general body massage and by application of herbs and oils to the skin, particularly to the back near the region of the heart.

The channel to the stomach (visvodhara) can be treated by massage of the abdomen, around the navel, as well as by applying herbs and oils to the navel (like ginger paste). Herbs for the digestive system are another method.

The reproductive channel (kuhu) can be treated by massage of the perineum or the point above the penis, as well as by oil application to the urethra (in women also). Brahmi oil is also good here for giving control of the sexual function.

The elimination channel (alambusha) can be treated by massage of the rectum or application of herbs and oils at this site. The alambusha is the next most important channel after the sushumna. Here vata is treated by medicated enemas (*basti*).

The channels can be treated through the senses, organs of action or systems of the body that apply to them, as well as by treating the chakras from which they branch off. A good method is to visualize these channels and direct the flow of prana through them via thought, viewing the prana as red or orange in color. Learning to visualize the nadis and the flow of energy through them is an important method of pranayama and pratyahara. The channels can also be treated through pranayama in which the flow of prana is directed along them via visualization. Note this in the chapter on pranayama.

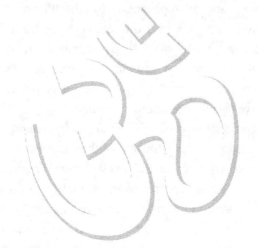

PART THREE

The Practices of Yoga and Ayurveda

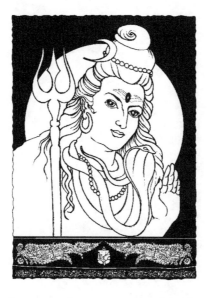

Techniques of Inner Transformation

Note that this section describes various practices relative to the doshic types of vata, pitta and kapha. If one is a combination of these types the rule to remember is to treat the dosha that is currently out of balance.

12

Yogic and Ayurvedic Diets

Similarities and Differences

And he knew that food was Brahman.
From food all beings are born,
by food they live and into food they return.

TAIITIRIYA UPANISHAD 3.2

Food, *anna*, is the first Sanskrit word for Brahman, the Supreme Godhead. Everything in the universe is food. The inner Self, Atman, is the eater of the food which is everything. All that we see is food for the soul. Our development as a soul depends upon our ability to eat and digest the food that is our life. Food, anna, is the basis of life, prana. It carries the life-force and sustains it in the body.

The type of food that we seek reflects our level of development. From the nature of the food that a person chooses, his or her stage of consciousness is revealed. Yoga and Ayurveda emphasize a pure vegetarian or what is called a sattvic diet — a diet to encourage the development of sattva, the higher qualities of peace, love and awareness. Eating is our first interaction with our environment. If that is not based upon love and compassion, all our other actions are bound to suffer.

Ayurveda emphasizes right diet as the foundation of all healing therapies. Food is the first and most important form of medicine. Without right food no other healing modality can be effective. Ayurveda recommends sattvic or pure food because sattva creates balance, eliminates harmful factors and helps reduce all the doshas.

The basis of sattva is the attitude of ahimsa (non-harming). Sattvic diet is first of all vegetarian, avoiding any products that involve killing or harming of animals. Sattvic diet additionally emphasizes natural foods, foods grown in harmony with nature, on good soils, ripened naturally, cooked in the right manner and with the right attitude of love. Such foods are carriers of prana and consciousness.

Yogis are among the strictest people in the world about their diets. Not only are they vegetarian, they avoid commercially prepared food, fried food, and fast food. They refrain from eggs and garlic as well. Yogis commonly cook their own food or travel with their own cooks, who know the art of sattvic cooking. If you invite such a real yogi over to your house, he or she may show you how to cook, probably first going to the store and making sure to have all the right food articles and then preparing a wonderful meal that becomes almost a sacrament.

However, a yogic diet has a different purpose than an ayurvedic diet and the two should not simply be equated. This reflects the different purposes of the two disciplines: Ayurveda aims at bringing health and balance to the physical body; yoga aims at helping us transcend body consciousness. While Ayurveda works to improve bodily health, yoga helps us move beyond bodily limitations. For this reason, most traditional yogic disciplines are ascetic in nature, including fasting and light diet, raw foods and detoxification measures, as well as sensory deprivation, pranayama and meditation. All these factors not only tend to reduce physical consciousness but can aggravate vata, which represents the airy or non-physical component of our nature. Traditional Ayurveda, on the other hand, emphasizes cooked foods, nutritive diet, and protecting ourselves from the elements in order to build physical strength and prevent the doshas, particularly vata, from accumulating.

Raw or Cooked Foods

A lot of confusion exists today about the role of raw food diets in yoga and Ayurveda, and in vegetarianism in general. Some people identify vegetarian diet with raw food only. Cooking vegetables does not turn them into meat! Vegetarian diet includes all non-meat food products, even those which are cooked. Many food items, like rice or potatoes, have to be cooked in order to become digestible.

Ayurveda generally does not recommend raw food diets for long term health maintenance but only for short term detoxification. This is because raw food is harder to digest and does not provide as much bulk nutrition as cooked food. Ayurveda recommends specific diets to counter our dosha. These are based mainly on whole grains, beans, root vegetables, seeds and nuts, with only secondary amounts of raw food items — what could be called "balanced" or "nutritive" vegetarian diets.

This ayurvedic view that cooked food is better, however, has caused some people to think that raw food is bad from an ayurvedic perspective. Because of the connection between Ayurveda and yoga, these individuals may consider that raw food diets are unyogic. However, if we look at traditional yogic texts we do find an emphasis on raw food. Yogic diet is traditionally called a diet of fruits and roots (*phala mula*), though it includes grains and dairy products as well. Yogis in retreat in nature live on wild food as part of their spiritual regimen and as a means of connecting with the forces of nature.

Raw foods, we should note, increase the air and ether elements in the body and mind, the vata components. Cooked foods are better for increasing earth and water elements, the kapha components, and also for increasing fire, the pitta factor. This makes cooked foods easier to digest and better to build the body, but raw food better for promoting our subtle sensitivities of prana and mind.

A yogic diet emphasizes the development of air and ether elements, not only for detoxification but also for opening the mind, whose nature is mainly air and ether. For this reason it recommends raw foods as well as fasting. Reducing the body allows the mind to develop and expand, lowering our body consciousness and increasing detachment.

Yogic diet considers not only the role of the doshas, which is the main factor in ayurvedic diet, but the role of prana. Raw foods are rich in prana, which the yogi is seeking to develop as the higher energy of the mind. Raw food bring the pranic force not only into the body but into the mind as well. Raw food is part of a traditional yogic diet for cleansing of the nadis or the channels, which occurs through increasing prana. Great yogis were said to be able to live on the air or prana alone. Others could live on only water, yet others on a little fruit, milk or ghee only.

The yogic strategy is to increase agni (the digestive fire) through internal practices so that vata does not get aggravated in the practice of yoga. The correct practice of yoga, particularly pranayama, increases agni so that we are able to digest raw foods. With a higher internal heat we are not so dependent upon heat in our food and do better with a cooling diet. The yogi with a stronger digestive and pranic fire can handle raw foods, temperature extremes and other physical imbalances that ordinarily cause disease. Ayurveda, however, aims at the ordinary person who requires protection from these external vicissitudes and harsher aspects of life.

However, those of us who are only part-time yogis, and rarely ascetics, may not have the digestive power to handle raw food items, particularly for long periods of time. This is especially true of vata types who usually have a weak or variable digestive power. They must remember the vata-aggravating potential of a traditional yogic diet. But kapha people with their low digestive fire and slow metabolism can be weakened by too much raw food as well. Even pitta types will find raw food too light to sustain long-term energy and vitality, particularly if they are engaged in strenuous physical activity.

Yet most people can benefit from periodic raw food diets for detoxification purposes, particularly in late springtime, April or May depending upon the climate, which is the natural season for detoxification. We also require some amount of raw food in our diets, generally about ten or twenty percent, to afford the proper vitamins, minerals and enzymes that abound in these foods. Good raw food items to take with meals are cucumbers, radishes, carrots, tomatoes, and various types of sprouts, cilantro and parsley.

In addition, those who want to cleanse not only the physical body but the subtle body can do so with the aid of raw food diets combined with asana, pranayama, mantra and meditation. Such a practice can be done for one to three months depending upon one's constitution. Anyone who seriously wants to go into yoga practice should consider such preliminary detoxification approaches, particularly as allied with the ayurvedic detoxification program of pancha karma. As most people in the West are overweight and have many toxins in their systems, these detoxification methods are often the first measures in reclaiming health.

To avoid the danger of over detoxification with raw foods there is a simple test. Raw food diets should not serve to suppress our digestive fire, leaving us without a healthy appetite to sustain us. Along with the raw food diet, try to follow a regimen to increase the digestive fire with the use of spices like ginger, cayenne, cinnamon and basil, or the ayurvedic formula *trikatu*. One should only take raw food to the extent that one's digestive fire has the capacity. Nevertheless, the importance of raw food for purification should not be overlooked. As one advances in spiritual practices, one can handle more raw food and require less and less food.

Advanced yogis naturally gravitate toward raw foods, as well as grains and dairy products. They prefer living on pranic foods to anything processed or overcooked, and may ultimately give up cooked food altogether. Seeing nature as their mother, they dislike commercially prepared or grown food. Spiritual progress reflects a growing sensitivity to food and requires food that contains both prana and love as the main ingredients.

Yoga, Meat and Ahimsa

Meat-eating is something that any student of yoga should reduce, if not avoid altogether. This is particularly true of red meat. Of course, the main reason is that meat-eating violates the yogic principle of ahimsa or non-violence, which is the first of the yamas or lifestyle disciplines of yoga practice. If our yoga practice is based upon harming other creatures it cannot go far.

The human body, teeth and digestive system are that of a vegetarian animal. Vegetable foods provide the ideal nutrition to build up our human sensitivities through a refined physical and astral body. We cannot readily break down animal tissues into the right components for human tissue. Instead of digesting and transforming meat into the appropriate human tissue, its animal energies are preserved and become substituted for our human tissues.

Meat increases the animal fire in the body, bringing the samskaras or tendencies of carnivorous animals to function within us. This promotes anger, lust and fear and other negative emotions. The flame created by a meat diet is impure and projects an emotional smoke that distorts the mind and the nervous system. Meat diet communicates the energy of destruction to the cells, which in turn promotes processes of disease and decay within them. It brings in a subtle energy of death into the auric field, reducing the flow of higher pranas into the body. The lives of the creatures we have eaten weigh down the astral body with their negative feelings and impressions.

Meat produces a heavy or tamasic type of tissue that clogs the channels and tends to make the mind dull. This does not mean that spiritual practices will have no effect for a meat eater but that if these are successful, which is less likely, there is a danger that the meat in the system, which is a crude form of fuel, may cause the person to overheat or create a kind of smoke that distorts any higher experiences. Not only violence and crime but religious intolerance has historically been more common among meat-eating groups. This is not just a moral but an energetic issue for body, mind and spirit on both individual and collective levels. If we add the damage that meat consumption is doing to the planet through the destruction of the rain forests, pollution of land and water, and the increasing difficulty of sustaining a meat diet for an ever-growing human population, then the magnitude of this problem cannot be glossed over. We cannot truly evolve as a species and go beyond war and crime until we give up eating our animal brothers and sisters.

Many people today are not strict vegetarians but eat chicken and fish as well. While this animal flesh is less harmful than red meat, it is still the life of another living and moving creature. Not only are these food articles harmful for yogic practice, they are harmful for the planet and for other creatures. The amount of chickens raised today in factory farms is in the many billions.

Other vegetarians eat eggs, so-called lacto-ovo vegetarians. Even vegetarians who do not eat whole eggs may consume many eggs in other food products. Eggs are common ingredients in breads, pastries, noodles, mayonnaise, and salad dressings. Avoiding eggs can be difficult, even if one does not take them directly. One must carefully look at the label of foods to see if eggs are included. While eating eggs causes less harm than eating fish, chicken or red meat, eggs are still animal flesh and cause exploitation to these creatures. Many Hindu temples do not allow those who eat eggs into their inner sanctuaries. The complications of factory farming and genetic engineering to chickens and eggs are other reasons to avoid them.

Unfortunately, many yoga students and even yoga teachers in the West partake of meat diets, sometimes serving chicken and fish at yoga or meditation retreats. How this can be ignored, given the dharmic traditions of ahimsa, is hard to understand, particularly when vegetarian items are easy to get.

The Modern Dilemma: The Era of Bad Food

Right diet is not just a question of food type but food quality. The quality of food in our culture is generally low, as most of us have come to know. If food is God, then our God is certainly dead, or at least he has become little more than a business arrangement for maximum profit! Our food is mass produced, mass prepared and mass consumed, with little care or attention and certainly little love or consciousness. Poor food quality begins with bad soils, chemical fertilizers, and the use of insecticides and herbicides on the plants, the long term effects of which are unknown. Poor food quality is compounded by premature picking, artificial ripening, long transportation and refrigeration that often eliminates whatever real vitality managed to survive in the plant. On top of this comes the processing of food, which may include irradiation, freezing and canning, along with additives and preservatives of all types. As if this was not enough, our cooking procedures involve microwave ovens, over-cooking, and an excess use of oils, sugar, salt and spices. The result is that we don't so much eat our food as our food eats us, providing not so much nourishment as a breeding ground for toxins.

Yet however bad this situation may be, it is likely to get worse. Genetic engineering is now adding genes from bacteria, viruses, other plants and animals to food crops. Even the seeds that we use to grow our plants are becoming genetically modified. There are bacteria, nut and flower genes in soybeans. Fish and pig genes are being added to tomatoes. The main reason for such changes is to make the food look better, last longer, or become more resistant to herbicides and pesticides so that these can be used more abundantly, not to actually make the food more nutritious.

Such genetic changes are unlikely to be mentioned on la-bels. Already most of the soybeans grown are genetically engi-neered, making it difficult for vegetarians since soybeans are common in most vegetarian products. Naturally, for anyone trying to follow a pure yogic diet, such changes are distressing. Since we cannot avoid eating and, if we travel at all, may be forced to eat out, we can only hope to reduce the amount of bad food that we consume.

This modern food dilemma is forcing all of us to become more conscious of our diets. We must learn to grow our own food, to support local and organic gardeners, and to become politically active on environmental matters. Food is the sacred root of life. If we compromise it we are only jeopardizing our own health and happiness. Unfortunately the coming century stands to inherit not only bad food, but bad water and bad air as well. We can at least get good bottled water. The air and

food are more precarious. Therefore, raising our food consciousness and food discrimination is an important part of any eco-
logical strategy for saving the planet.

A true yogi should be among those in the forefront working for protection of animals and protection of the Earth. If we
act now there is still much that we can do to improve if not
fundamentally alter these negative conditions. The Earth itself,
like the human body, has tremendous powers of revitalization
if we learn to facilitate this healing force to operate without our
obstruction.

Dairy Products and Yoga

The yoga traditions of India regard dairy products as excellent foods, particularly for individuals on the spiritual path.
While dairy is not recommended for all types, particularly not
for kaphas, it has an important role not only for maintaining
health but for promoting longevity. Ancient Vedic civilization
grew up around the cow, which provided milk, cream, butter,
and yogurt. Throughout history, these foods have been favor-
ites of the yogis who did not find dairy products harmful to
their health. In his childhood, the great avatar Krishna was no-
torious for helping himself to the freshly churned butter any
unsuspecting housewife left unattended.

Ayurveda uses dairy preparations medicinally, particularly
for improving resistance to disease, and to promote convalescence and regeneration. These include milk decoctions, medicated butters and ghees (clarified butter). Dairy is not only recommended for the young, but for the elderly and for anyone
who is debilitated or needing strength. Many yogis take to a
predominantly milk diet for extended periods of time. Freshly
boiled milk, with spices and raw sugar, is considered to be an
excellent food.

However, this depends upon good quality milk from cows

who have been treated well, which takes us back to our modern dilemma. Such milk is rarely available commercially. Otherwise, poorly prepared dairy products from badly treated cows increases mucus in the system and promotes food and sinus allergies and candida.

There are a number of health issues relating to milk products that we must understand in order to use dairy correctly. Some people lack the enzymes necessary to digest dairy products because their ethnic group has no history of taking dairy. Adults who weren't breast-fed as children may also have trouble with it. Other problems arise not from dairy products themselves but from their improper preparation. Just as whole wheat flour is quite different from bleached white flour, so naturally-prepared dairy products are quite distinct from dairy products commonly sold in supermarkets.

In India the cow is allowed to give its milk to its calf first. Only the leftover milk, which is often considerable, is taken by humans. If the calf is taken away from its mother, her milk loses much of its nourishing quality. The dairy industry removes calves from their mothers and slaughters them. We kill the animal's child and then drink its milk. How would a human mother feel under such circumstances? When a cow hears the call of her calf, she immediately begins to secrete milk. The cow knows when her calf is going to be killed, and her distress causes toxins to be secreted into her milk.

Cows are mistreated in many other ways, including being confined to pens and milked by machines. They are now hybrid animals, produced through artificial insemination, genetically redesigned to produce far more milk than is healthy for them to do. They are fed hormones, antibiotics and inorganic grains. Chemical residues are absorbed into their tissues and concentrated in their milk. Pasteurization, homogenization and long term refrigeration of dairy products also weaken their benefits.

Ayurvedic texts explains the properties of various dairy products in great detail. They tell us that the quality of meat or dairy products from tethered or confined animals is much less than that from animals who are able to graze freely. Hence we cannot equate modern factory farm dairy products with those of ayurvedic texts. Clearly we should try to get raw or organic dairy products, or be careful in using dairy products at all.

Of dairy products, milk and ghee are excellent for the practice of yoga. Milk is best taken freshly boiled with spices like ginger, cinnamon and cardamom. Yogurt is better if mixed with water and made into a drink (Indian buttermilk or *lassee*). Otherwise it is a bit heavy and mucus -forming, not the weight-reducing food it is thought to be.

Most cheeses are made with rennet that comes from cow intestines. Strict vegetarians therefore only use cheese that has been produced with vegetarian enzymes. Such cheeses are now available in most natural food stores. Also cottage cheese, cream cheese and farmer's cheese (Indian *paneer*) are very good.

Yoga and Spices

As most Indian cooking is very spicy, some people assume that a yogic diet must have a lot of spices, including much cayenne or chilies. This is not the case. People raised on high spice diets, like those raised in India, can tolerate more of these, even on a yogic diet. However, a yogic diet should not be too spicy because most spices are rajasic and irritate the nerves. It should emphasize sweet spices like ginger, cinnamon, cardamom, basil and fennel, which are sattvic.

Many spicy foods, particularly in restaurants, are prepared with bad oils. This is not a good combination. If you take a high spice diet you should make sure that you are using good quality natural spices along with good quality natural oils like ghee. Good ghee should be used, produced from raw or organic butter rather than from regular commercial butter.

Yoga and Sugar

Some people are of the opinion that any spiritual diet should avoid sugar altogether. This is mainly owing to the dangers caused by white sugar. White sugar is a processed and refined food and should be avoided for this reason. Yet we all require a certain amount of natural sugars, like honey or unrefined sugar (*jaggary*) in the diet. This is particularly true in the case of children. So too, as the kundalini develops through spiritual practice, pure sugars may be required to keep the metabolism in balance. For this reason natural sweets in moderation are part of a yogic diet.

Sattvic Diet

To follow a sattvic diet we must understand the six tastes. Sweet is the primary sattvic taste because it is nourishing, balancing and agreeable to the mind and senses. However, by sweet taste Ayurveda means natural sweets, not processed sugars, much less artificial sweeteners. It includes sugars, starches, carbohydrates and oils, such as those found in fruit, grains, vegetables, seeds and nuts.

Pungent, sour and salty tastes tend to be rajasic because they are stimulating in properties. While this makes them good for improving digestion and other therapeutic qualities, it makes them potentially irritating to the nervous system. Pungent or spicy taste has a hot and expansive nature that can push our energies too far if used in excess, causing depletion. Salt can clog the arteries and channels because of its mineral content, like the salts that corrode plumbing pipes. Sour taste, like alcohol, can promote fermentation in the body.

Bitter and astringent tastes tend to be tamasic because their long term reducing effects, which, however useful for detoxification and weight reduction, have potential side effects. Bitter taste, with its cold and light properties, has a detoxifying effect that weakens agni and aggravates vata (causing nervousness). Astringent taste, which is constricting, can result in the retention of waste materials, and also increases vata.

Yet each taste can be sattvic, rajasic or tamasic depending on how it is used. It is a question of proportions. We need the right balance of all six tastes. This consists of a predominately sweet taste diet, with the use of pungent, salty, and sour articles as condiments, and the use of bitter and astringent tastes for detoxification as necessary.

THE SIX TASTES

Taste	Element	Dosha	Guna
Sweet	earth and water	VP- K+	Sattva
Salty	water and fire	V- KP+	Rajas
Sour	earth and fire	V- KP+	Rajas
Pungent	fire and air	K- PV+	Rajas
Bitter	air and ether	PK- V+	Tamas
Astringent	earth and air	PK- V+	Tamas

Too much sweet food, even of a natural type, becomes tamasic or dulling and can clog the channels. Artificially prepared or processed sweets tend to do this in any quantity. Sweet spices, like ginger, cinnamon and mint are sattvic, as is sour fruit like lemon and lime. Some bitter herbs, like gotu kola, are sattvic because bitter taste with its air and ether elements helps expand the mind. Overeating of any food type can become tamasic and cause stagnation. On the other hand, undereating or taking a too light or too stimulating diet increases rajas. Only the right diet and proper food quantity is sattvic. Sattvic diet is pleasant but evenly balanced in taste, containing some amount of all six tastes and only taken in the amount necessary to fill half the stomach.

Sattvic Diets for the Doshas

Ayurveda prescribes dietary regimens for the different doshas. In this regard, three tastes decrease and three tastes increase each of the doshas as described in the table above. A number of good ayurvedic cookbooks exist for those interested in going into this matter in more detail.[28]

Ayurvedic cooking and dietetic approaches are mainly concerned with physical health and do not always address the issue of sattva. Hence they may discuss certain food types that are not sattvic in nature. Yoga, on the other hand, emphasizing a sattvic diet, may include foods that can aggravate certain doshas. For an optimal dietary regimen one should combine a sattvic diet with a diet appropriate for one's doshic type. Abundant sattvic foods exist for all constitutions. One can take the list of sattvic foods given below and adjust it relative to the foods for one's constitution.

Sattvic diet is a matter of timing of meals as well as food type. One should avoid heavy or mucus-producing food in the morning or in the evening as it is more likely to clog the system at these times. The morning meal should be light and stimulating. The main meal should be at noon, followed by a period of rest or relaxation, or in the early evening. Eating late at night, except some light food like fruit or milk, weighs the body and mind down.

One should also remember the particular imbalances that are likely through yogic practices. As yogic practices like pranayama and meditation are more likely to aggravate vata, so vata-pacifying foods must be considered relative to these practices. Note also the information on ojas in the earlier chapter on prana, tejas and ojas. An ojas-increasing diet is important for many yogic approaches.

Pranic Diet

Yogic diet is not simply a sattvic diet but a pranic diet, full of the vital force needed to energize the mind and subtle body. In this regard different foods relate to the different pranas.

Of the five pranas, pranic foods are mainly green leafy vegetables and sprouts that grow quickly, particularly in the springtime when prana is abundant. These are stimulating, cooling and purifying. Raw food diets with many chlorophyll dominant foods and herbs promote prana, particularly if combined with mild aromatic spices like ginger, coriander or mint.

Apanic foods are foods that grow beneath the earth, mainly root vegetables like potatoes, carrots and sweet potatoes. They includes mushrooms, which arise out of the earth. Such foods increase strength, endurance and ojas but can be a little heavy. As the soul or jiva in plants dwells in the ground, roots can contain great vital energy. This category includes special powerful root herbs like ginseng or *shatavari*, including tonics to the reproductive system, which is ruled by apana.

Samana foods are mainly whole grains which have a balancing effect (when well tolerated), particularly rice. This is why whole grains should be the foundation of most diets. Dairy products, which are predigested foods, come under samana as well, as does honey and raw sugars. Such foods are nourishing but not heavy, unless taken in excess, and easy to digest.

Vyana foods are those which spread on the ground like squash, melons, strawberries, tomatoes and beans. These are strengthening and stimulating and help our energy expand. They are usually taken along with grains or samana foods.

Udana foods are fruit and nuts that grow above in trees. They contain more of the ether element and nourish the deeper mind and heart. They can be taken by themselves and are very wholesome, light and balancing.

Yoga emphasizes foods with sattvic prana. This is most commonly found in foods produced above the ground like fruit and nuts. Foods that grow on the ground, like tomatoes or strawberries, have a tendency to develop rajas. Food that grow or develop from beneath the ground tend to tamas, like garlic, onions and mushrooms. But these are only secondary factors. Sattvic roots and vegetables are quite common as well.

Yogic diet consists primarily of udana-type foods, like fruit, to help make our prana rise, and samana foods, like rice and milk, to keep us in balance, but food for the other pranas is also good. We should make sure to have foods for all the five pranas as well as all six tastes.

While taking pranic foods one must be careful to keep one's doshas in balance. Vata types need nourishing food that strengthens apana and so require more root vegetables or root herbs. All doshic types benefit from foods that relate to samana, like whole grains, which are balancing in nature. In addition, spices may be required to strengthen the digestive fire and the fire of prana (pranagni), particularly if one's diet is mainly cold in nature like pranic foods tend to be. Prana dominates in air and ether elements and so needs the heat of fire, the grounding of earth, and the moistening quality of water to keep it in balance.

Good Foods for Yoga Practice

- Fruit of all types, particularly of a sweet nature, taken fresh and whole
- All vegetables, except too much onions and garlic
- Whole grains of all types, particularly rice, wheat and oats
- Beans in moderation, except those that are not too heavy in properties, like mung, aduki or tofu

- Nuts and seeds like almond, coconut, walnuts, pecans, and sesame, yet not overly roasted or salted
- Good natural plant-based oils of all types like sesame, olive and sunflower, also butter and ghee (clarified butter)
- Dairy products from cows who have been treated well, particularly milk, ghee, yogurt and cottage cheese
- Natural sugars like raw sugar (jaggery), honey, maple syrup, and molasses
- Sweet spices like ginger, cinnamon, cardamom, fennel, cumin, coriander, turmeric, mint, basil, fenugreek
- Herbal teas, natural water, and fruit juices (particularly water with lemon or lime)
- Food prepared with love and consciousness

Foods to Reduce or Avoid

- Meat and fish of all types, including eggs
- Artificial, processed and junk food of all types
- Canned food, except naturally canned fruit and tomatoes
- Poor quality oils, animal fats and margarine
- Dairy products from factory farms
- Garlic, onions and overly spicy food
- Fried food of all types
- White sugar and white flour
- Artificial sweeteners and condiments
- Any overly cooked foods, old, stale or recooked food
- Alcohol, tobacco or other stimulants
- Tap water or any artificial beverages
- Any irradiated food articles, microwave cooking
- Genetically engineered food items
- Food taken in a disturbed environment or eaten too quickly

13

Preparing Soma

Herbs for the Practice of Yoga

Plants who are Queens of the Soma, manifold,
with a hundredfold perceptive power. I take you as
the best for the fulfillment of the heart's desire.
Plants who are Queens of the Soma, spread over all
the Earth, generated by the Divine Father,
may you impart vigor to this herb.

RIG VEDA X.97.18-19

Herbs are powerful aids in the practice of yoga. They are useful not only for treating diseases and for rejuvenation but for awakening all our higher faculties. Anyone involved in yoga should consider taking helpful herbs on a regular basis. Yogis commonly have taken herbs to aid in their practice and to stimulate both prana and the higher mind.

Many of the oriental tonic herbs becoming popular in this country today, like ginseng and *ashwagandha*, are excellent for yoga practice because they increase our deeper vital energies (chi or prana). Such herbs possess overall strengthening properties for the muscles and nerves, especially helpful for vegetarians who may need a deeper form of nutrition. But even commonly available herbs and spices like ginger, turmeric or licorice have value for yoga practice. Herbs are important adjuncts that can catalyze processes that otherwise may be difficult to achieve.

We can all benefit from a daily usage of herbs. Our daily herbs may be as important as our daily bread. The effects of herbs, however, do not manifest immediately. Like food, the benefits from herbs accrue over time and require the right diet and lifestyle regimens to support them. For this reason, we must give herbs the proper circumstances in which to work and not simply treat them like drugs. Note that this chapter will not discuss the background of ayurvedic herbology, the preparation of herbs or related issues. These can be found in other books on Ayurveda.[29] We will focus on relevant herbs for yoga practice.

Herbs and Soma

According to the Vedic view, the sap of herbs contains an powerful life essence called soma. The soma from plants can combine with ojas, which is the soma or life-essence of the body, and boost it to a higher level of activity. This healing essence of plants reacts with the plasma (*rasa*) in the body, creating a superior form of plasma to nurture and rejuvenate other tissues. It creates an exhilarating effect that promotes healing and transformative processes on all levels.

Some botanists have looked for an original soma plant, as if soma was only a single herb. They are making a mistake. Vedic texts mention many different types of soma plants, and soma is the essence of all plants. They commonly equate soma with honey (*madhu*), which itself is produced from the essence of plants through their pollen. Soma, therefore, refers to various special essences (*soma rasas*) that are found more in some plants than others but exist throughout the plant kingdom.

Classical ayurvedic texts like the *Susruta Samhita* mention twenty-four soma plants and eighteen soma-like plants.[30] The *Atharva Veda*[31] mentions, among soma-producing plants, grains like barley, herbs likes *durva* and nervines like cannabis (*bhang*). Kushta (Saussurea lappa) is another plant commonly mentioned along with soma.[32] Ephedra (Ma huang) has been used as a soma substitute, particularly by the ancient Persians who followed a similar religion to the Vedic Hindus. Soma is a general plant essence, not a particular species. Soma-type ingredients are most common in tonic and nervine herbs. Traditionally in India, various members of the lily and orchid family were used for this purpose because of their strong nutritive and nervine properties and their abundant juice.

Soma ingredients are most prevalent among plants growing in the mountains, particularly by streams and lakes. Kashmir and its Manasa (Dal) lake, the upper Indus around Ladakh, and Mount Kailas and Lake Manasarovar in Tibet were considered to be the best soma regions. High altitudes impart a special prana to plants that allows them to transmit cosmic and astral influences that are more accessible in mountain regions. Any mountain-grown plants tend to have more soma or vital juice. This is well known in most native healing traditions.

Soma is a very volatile substance, however. It is found mainly in wild plants, freshly picked. Ayurveda always considers that the fresh juice of the plant has the strongest healing properties. This is because it contains the most soma. Even plants that contain soma ingredients can lose these if they are not taken fresh or prepared so as to endure. This is an important issue in herbalism today because wild plants are hard to get and it is also hard to preserve their potency. In terms of soma, the quality of herbs is as important as their specific nature.

Soma plants were prepared by first crushing the juice. This was then mixed or cooked with milk, ghee, yogurt, barley, honey or sugar cane juice and sometimes fermented, as many different types of soma preparations existed. They were sometimes prepared with metals like gold, just as ayurvedic herbs in India are today. Such alchemical somas were the basis of later alchemical and tantric medicines. Soma was designed to transform the base metal of our worldly nature to the gold of spirituality. This is not just a symbol. The base metal is the physical body; the gold is the purified subtle body. Soma was used to help awaken and energize the subtle body. Some soma preparations were used for spiritual purposes, some for healing purposes and some for both.

Plants also contain a special form of agni or the vegetable fire that allows them to digest light through photosynthesis. The agni of plants, which are pranic creatures, connects to pranagni, the agni of prana in the human body, warming and stimulating the life-force. Generally, spicy herbs with their naturally hot potency contain more agni energy, particularly spicy nervines like calamus, *pippali* or *shankha pushpi*. The combination of herbs high in agni and herbs high in soma works well for inner development. Agni-dominant herbs help purify, extract and digest soma herbs.

There are as many forms of soma as there are of agni. Each kosha has its own soma or nectar, which is the best type of food for it. Herbs provide soma for the body and prana, creating a special brain secretion that promotes contentment and nourishes the higher brain centers. This secretion is reflected as a certain form of saliva produced during pranayama.

The soma essence of plants is better transmitted if herbs are prepared along with ritual, mantra and meditation, which create a vehicle for the astral energy of the plant. Mantra is another form of agni that helps catalyze the soma ingredients in plants.

Herbs and Prana

Herbs mainly work at the level of pranamaya kosha, the vital energy or pranic body. Their effect is at a subtler level than food and at a heavier level than mental and sensory influences.

Herbs therefore link body and mind together via the prana. They stimulate the flow of prana through the channels and nadis. The subtle body itself with its various chakras is like a tree with different branches. Herbs facilitate movement of energy through this plant. They work to catalyze pranic processes both of growth and elimination. They aid prana in its job of keeping us healthy, strong, and aware.

Herbs for the Body and Hatha Yoga

All herbs that deal with physical health issues have some potential use in yoga practice. Here we will focus on the most important types, which are those that aid in asana practice.

1. Herbs to increase flexibility, promote circulation and stimulate the movement of energy. Such herbs aid in the proper performance of asanas by improving musculoskeletal function and coordination. They are usually classified as anti-rheumatic or anti-arthritic agents. They are mainly herbs for hatha yoga.

Typical herbs: *guggul, shallaki, myrrh, nirgundi, turmeric, saffron, Siberian ginseng, angelica, kava kava, dasha mula (ayurvedic formula).*

These are usually taken with honey and warm water or with spicy stimulants like ginger and cinnamon to increase their effects. They do better if supplemented with oil massage, particularly with medicated sesame oil formulas, or with sweating therapies and saunas.

2. Herbs to increase physical energy and vitality. They strengthen ojas and through it promote soma, which is the higher form of ojas or our vital essence. They are usually tonic and rejuvenative agents, with strong nutritive properties, strengthening also the reproductive system. They build stamina and endurance, af-

fording steadiness in yoga postures and in pranayama.

Typical herbs: *ashwagandha, amalaki, shatavari, bala, vidari, ginseng, dioscorea, kapikacchu, lotus seeds, licorice, saw palmetto, fo ti.*

These are usually taken with milk, raw sugar, ghee and other nutritive items to boost their strengthening powers. They combine well with raw (unheated) honey, particularly if it is fresh (less than six months old). They are best taken along with a nutritive vegetarian diet (like the anti-vata diet). A few spices should be added to them, like ginger and cinnamon, to aid in their digestion as they tend to be heavy.

3. Herbs for cooling and cleansing the body. These herbs remove toxins from the blood, the tissues and internal organs. They are usually bitter or astringent in taste and may contain large amounts of chlorophyll.

Typical herbs: *aloe gel, guduchi, gentian, barberry, gotu kola, brahmi, plantain, dandelion, comfrey leaf, nettles, yarrow, yellow dock.*

These herbs are taken with ghee, aloe gel, honey and other reducing agents. They are often combined with raw food diets, green juices, and other detoxification measures.

Herbs for the Five Pranas

The key to healing at an inner level is keeping the five pranas moving properly. Herbs aid in this process. Below are typical herbs for stimulating the five pranas. Some herbs are good for more than one prana. These categories overlap somewhat the herbs for body and mind, because prana works on both levels.

Prana: Spicy diaphoretic herbs that increase our power of inhalation, open the head and sinuses, stimulate the mind and senses, and improve the appetite: cinnamon, sage, calamus, mint, thyme, tulsi, eucalyptus, ephedra, cloves, pippali, shilajit.

Apana: Mild laxative herbs that increase elimination and cleanse the downward channels, aiding in the absorption of Prana through the large intestine: triphala, haritaki, psyllium, flax seed, castor oil, aloe gel, cascara sagrada, asafoetida, hingashtak (ayurvedic formula).

Samana: Spicy herbs that aid in digestion and absorption through the small intestine: cardamom, fennel, ginger, cayenne, mustard, cumin, basil, black pepper, nutmeg, trikatu (ayurvedic formula).

Vyana : Spicy and bitter herbs that promote circulation both through the heart, the blood and the musculoskeletal system: cinnamon, nirgundi, arjuna, elecampane, guggul, saffron, turmeric, guduchi, Siberian ginseng, angelica, kava kava.

Udana: Mainly spicy and astringent herbs that strengthen the voice and stop cough, as well as increase vitality and power of effort. Many herbs for prana work here as well, particularly those that stop cough: calamus, bayberry, elecampane, lobelia, tulsi, haritaki, peppermint, mullein, vasa, coltsfoot, cherry bark, licorice.

Herbs for the Mind and Meditation

Many herbs possess nervine properties and action on the mind. They can be divided into several main categories and have a usage for the higher yogas.

1. Herbs to stimulate the mind and senses and improve perception. These open the channels, increase cerebral circulation and remove mucus from the head. They increase perception

and discrimination, facilitating the process of insight and meditation. They are similar to herbs to move prana.

Typical herbs: *calamus, tulsi, basil, pippali, bayberry, ephedra (ma huang), sage, elecampane.*

These herbs are taken along with warm water and honey (particularly honey that is older, which has more drying properties) to improve their effects. They are the main herbs used in nasya therapy.

2. Herbs to increase awareness and intelligence, strengthening in the mind. They are special tonic and building agents for the mind and nerve tissue, similar to the tonics for the body. They increase soma in the nervous system, helping us to gain concentration, contentment and joy and to overcome pain.

Typical herbs: *shankha pushpi, brahmi, gotu kola, ashwagandha, haritaki, shatavari, bala, kapikacchu, arjuna, lotus seeds, shilajit.*

These herbs, like the tonics for the body which they resemble, are usually taken along with warm milk, raw sugar, raw honey, ghee and other nutritive items to boost their strengthening powers.

3. Herbs for calming the mind. These are mild sedative and pain relieving agents, but also slow down the mind for meditation. They are less nutritive than the mind tonics and better for reducing anxiety and agitated nerves.

Typical herbs: *jatamamsi, valerian, nutmeg, passion flower, kava kava, scullcap, lady's slipper, zizyphus seeds.*

These herbs may be taken with other soothing agents like ghee or aloe gel to improve their calmative properties. Jatamamsi is regarded as the best.

Doshic Types and Yoga Practice

<u>Vata types</u>: suffer from lack of flexibility, dryness and stiffness,

and commonly develop arthritis. They benefit by herbs for improving flexibility, as well as by regular oil massage with sesame oil and its medicated varieties. Vatas also commonly suffer from low energy. They benefit by tonic herbs for improving energy, particularly ashwagandha.

Vata types have to be careful to keep apana balanced and often require a mild laxative like Triphala. However, since vata tends to disturb prana, herbs for the five pranas can be helpful for them, particularly pranic regulators like *tulsi* (holy basil). Vata people easily get ungrounded and unstable. They benefit by tonics of all types, particularly nervine tonics, along with herbs for calming the mind like jatamamsi and ashwagandha. They do best taking herbs with warm milk or with raw honey.

Pitta types: usually have internal heat and toxic blood that needs to be removed from the body for healing to occur. They benefit by cooling and detoxifying herbs like aloe gel, guduchi and barberry, along with green herbs and foods.

The mind itself is the seat of fire on a subtle level. Hence the mind and brain easily get overheated. Pittas need to keep their minds and emotions cool, avoiding emotions like anger that overheat the mind. For this, cooling-type nervines like gotu kola, brahmi, shatavari and jatamamsi are best. They do best taking herbs with milk or with aloe gel.

Kapha types: With their tendency towards stagnation, kapha types benefit by herbs to improve circulation, particularly guggul, myrrh and turmeric, which counter common kapha complaints like heart disease, diabetes, asthma and obesity. The best tonics for them are those that are not too heavy like shilajit, though they can benefit from ashwagandha or ginseng if their energy is very low.

Kapha, as mucus, blocks the channels and nadis of the head

and subtle body. They benefit from herbs to stimulate the mind and senses. For this, various spicy herbs are recommended, particularly calamus, ginger and pippali, along with the use of the neti pot and nasya therapy. As their prana easily becomes blocked by mucus, kaphas benefit from herbs for the five pranas, with the possible exception of the herbs for apana. They do best taking herbs with warm water or honey (over six months old).

Special Herbs for Yoga Practice

Below are listed special, mainly Indian herbs for yoga practice. These are available through many herb or ayurvedic stores. The herb is given along with its taste (rasa), heating effect (*virya*) and post-digestive action (*vipaka*). VPK is action on Vata, Pitta and Kapha: + is increasing, - is decreasing, = is balancing or neutral. For more information, including dosage and preparation, consult *Yoga of Herbs*.

Arjuna/ Terminalia arjuna

astringent/ cooling / pungent
PK- V+

Arjuna is a tonic and rejuvenative for the heart that promotes vyana vayu and increases prana. It helps develop devotion and gives us the extra courage and energy for our spiritual practice, just as Arjuna was able to fight for dharma at the side of Lord Krishna.

Amalaki/ Emblica officinalis

all tastes but salty/ cooling/sweet
VPK=

Amalaki is a tonic and rejuvenative for all the tissues. It balances the doshas and increases ojas. Taken in the form of a jelly called *Chyavan Prash,* it is an excellent food for yoga practice and a good energy booster. It is a prime tonic for young children, pregnant women, the elderly and anyone in need of extra strength and stamina.

Aloe Vera

> bitter, astringent, sweet/ cooling/ sweet
> PK- V+

Aloe is an entire medicine chest in itself. Relative to yoga practice, it is excellent for cleansing the plasma, skin, blood and the liver, all the main physical and pranic systems. It has rejuvenative effects for the female reproductive system as well.

Ashwagandha/ Withania somnifera

> bitter, sweet/ heating/ sweet
> VK- P+

Ashwagandha is the best ayurvedic tonic for both body and mind. It strengthens and nourishes the muscles, tendons, bones and nerves and builds ojas and tejas, fortifying the immune system. It is good for joint and nerve pain and is specific for lowering anxiety. It counters insomnia, calms the mind and promotes concentration, meditation and deep sleep. Ashwagandha is excellent in sports medicine for increasing endurance and protecting the bones and joints from injury.

Bayberry/ Myrica nagi

> pungent/ heating/ pungent
> KV- P+

Bayberry is an excellent herb for clearing kapha from the head and throat and for stimulating the mind and senses. It strengthens prana and udana and helps counter colds, flu and sore throat. It can be used with or as a substitute for calamus for clearing the head and sinuses.

Calamus/ Acorus calamus

pungent, bitter/ heating/ pungent
KV- P+

Calamus, also known as sweet flag, is a stimulant to the mind
and senses. It clears mucus from the head, throat and lungs. It
improves digestion, but in large dosages it becomes an emetic.
In Ayurveda it is mainly used to clear the subtle channels of
toxins, phlegm and blockages. Calamus increases the powers
of speech, reason and intelligence and sharpens discrimination.
It is excellent for mantra and meditation. It aids in spiritual
study and is said to increase knowledge of the higher Self.

Gotu Kola/ Brahmi

bitter, sweet, astringent/cooling/sweet
PK- V=

Brahmi is a close relative of gotu kola and is the preferable herb
but gotu kola can be used as a substitute when brahmi is not
available. Brahmi is a sedative, calmative, muscle relaxant and
pain-relieving agent. It has diuretic, hemostatic, and alterative
properties for toxic blood conditions and counters adrenal fatigue. It aids in controlling anger and attachment and for cooling and calming the mind. Its Sanskrit name, *brahmi*, reflects
its usage to promote knowledge of Brahman, the cosmic reality.

Brahmi and its relatives grows wild in many tropical areas,
including India and Hawaii. Brahmi juice taken in aloe juice is
an excellent detoxifying agent for body and mind. Prepared as a
medicated ghee, it is excellent for the liver and the nerves. Fresh
brahmi leaves preserved in raw honey is a good soma-producing agent.

Guduchi (Amrit)/ Tinospora cordifolia

bitter, astringent, sweet/ hot/ sweet

VPK=

Guduchi removes heat and toxins from a deep level of the tissues and nerves. It also cools and cleanses the mind. It is a rejuvenative for pitta and balances tejas. It is an excellent tonic for the immune system, particularly important for countering chronic low grade fevers or difficult infections from Epstein Barre virus to AIDS. It increases our positive energy in conditions of debility-like chronic fatigue syndrome.

Guggul/ Commiphora mukul

pungent, bitter, astringent, sweet/ heating/sweet
KV- P=

Guggul promotes flexibility of the muscles, ligaments and bones and is a prime medicine for arthritis. It also strengthens the heart, lowers cholesterol and prevents heart attacks. It keeps the blood clean and sattvic so it can vitalize all the tissues. Guggul regulates blood sugar and counters diabetes (a common disease of yogis whose metabolism can go through unusual fluctuations). It combines well with triphala as an excellent cleanser for the plasma and blood.

Jatamamsi/ Nardostachys jatamansi

bitter, astringent, sweet/ cooling/ sweet
VPK=

Jatamamsi is the best ayurvedic calmative herb, with soothing and strengthening properties for the brain and nervous tissue. It can be combined with ashwagandha as a brain tonic for vata and with cleansing agents like gotu kola for cooling the mind. Though related to valerian, it is a more balanced herb and easier to take. It improves our mental function and acuity rather than simply sedating it.

Kapikacchu/ Mucuna pruriens

bitter, sweet/ warm/ sweet
KV- P+

Kapikacchu is a powerful tonic herb strengthening both ojas and tejas and the deeper tissues of the nerve and reproductive systems. It calms vata, particularly in conditions of tremors or paralysis owing to debility. It is a natural source of L-dopa, useful in treating Parkinson's disease. A bean, it makes a pleasant and invigorating food taken along with rice.

Kava Kava/ Piper methysticum

pungent, bitter/ heating/ pungent
VK- P+

Kava kava improves circulation and relieves pain both to the musculoskeletal and nervous systems. It counters vata, promotes vyana, and facilitates rest, sleep and deep meditation. It helps promote a deep level of flexibility and detachment in both body and mind.

Myrrh/ Commiphora myrrha

bitter, pungent, astringent, sweet/ heating/ sweet
KV- P+

Myrrh, like guggul and shallaki, is excellent for promoting circulation to the muscles, joints and bones, for stopping pain and healing injuries. It also cleanses the blood and plasma and facilitates menstruation, strengthening the female reproductive system.

Nirgundi/ Vitex negundo

bitter, pungent/ heating/ pungent
VK- P+

Nirgundi is an excellent herb for ayurvedic massage oils and for steam therapy, stimulating vyana and vayu. It loosens toxins in the bones and joints and helps remove them from the body, countering pain and stiffness and reducing swelling. Useful with guggul and other herbs for improving flexibility and circulation.

Phyllanthus/ Phyllanthus niruri

bitter, astringent, sweet/ cooling/ pungent
VPK=

Phyllanthus is a tonic and rejuvenative herb for the liver and the blood and has been found useful in treating both chronic and acute hepatitis. It is good for deep-seated toxins in the organs that affect us on a subtle level and cause chronic diseases.

Prawal/ Red Coral Powder

sweet/cooling/sweet
PV- K+

Prawal is red coral powder, prepared either as an oxide (bhasma) or triturated through rose water (pishti). It has excellent properties for strengthening the bones, teeth, gums and hair. It counters pitta and builds ojas.

Sallaki/ Boswellia serrata

bitter, sweet, astringent/ cooling/ pungent
VPK=

Sallaki is a resin related to guggul and myrrh and used for similar purposes of cleansing the blood and countering arthritic pain and stiffness. It also aids in the healing of soft tissue injuries. Its cooling nature makes it particularly good for inflamed and swollen joints where there is pitta involvement.

Shankha Pushpi/ Evoluvus alsinodes

astringent / warm/ sweet
VPK=

Shankha pushpi is an excellent stimulant and tonic for the mind. It improves memory, concentration and perception, and aids in the rejuvenation of the brain. It stimulates our higher cerebral functions, improving our overall intelligence and creativity. *Sarasvata churna*, a powder prepared with this herb, is widely used in attention deficit disorder and helps prevent loss of memory.

Shatavari/ Asparagus racemosus

sweet, bitter/cooling/sweet
PV- K+

Shatavari is calming to the heart and increases love and devotion. Like ashwagandha, it is a prime tonic for all general usages but has a more specific action on the female system. It produces a higher quality plasma and guards against dehydration. It counters fever and acidity.

Shilajit

astringent, pungent, bitter/ warm/ pungent
KV- P+

Shilajit is a mineral pitch from the Himalayas and carries the healing power of these great mountains. Shilajit possesses great curative powers and is considered capable of treating many diseases, particularly those of the aging process. It is an important rejuvenative and tonic particularly for kapha, vata, and the kidneys, as in the case of people who have long suffered from diabetes and asthma. It can be taken for general health maintenance and is good for those who do much mental work or practice yoga.

Triphala

all tastes but salty/ neutral/ sweet
VPK=

Triphala, an important ayurvedic laxative formula, has an important usage in yoga. It controls the apana vayu, the downward moving air, and aids in the absorption of prana in the large intestine. It helps balance the metabolism and provides nutrition for the bones and nerves. Triphala facilitates the absorption of pure prana from our food, thus allowing for a more complete practice of pranayama or development of the life-force.

Tulsi (Holy Basil)/ Ocinum sanctum

pungent, sweet/ heating/ pungent
KV- P+

Tulsi is a form of basil that is an important herb for clearing the mind and brain and for increasing both wisdom and devotion. It promotes our higher pranas and is excellent for colds, flu, and sinus allergies. It is good to put a little tulsi in the water that one drinks.

Types of Ginseng

Siberian ginseng (Eleuthrococcus senticossus) is widely used for improving athletic performance, promoting elasticity of the joints and tendons, preventing injury during exercise and countering arthritis, particularly the chronic and degenerative type. These uses make it very helpful for asana practice.

Korean Ginseng builds chi (prana or the power of breath) and gives added endurance as well as increasing the overall adaptability of both body and mind. It promotes longevity and aids in rejuvenation. This makes it good for deeper yoga practices, but some people find it too stimulating and should be careful with it.

American ginseng may be preferable over the oriental as it is less likely to overheat the system. It helps prevent dehydration and is also a good antifatigue agent. It is good to take in the summer or for pitta constitutions.

Natural Soma Formula

ashwagandha, shatavari, kapikacchu, arjuna — 1 part each

brahmi, calamus, tulsi, licorice — 1/4 part each

Cook two tsps. of powdered herbs in two cups warm milk along with 1 tsp. raw sugar and 1 tsp. ghee. Take one cup in the morning and evening along with 1/4 tsp. of cardamom powder. Or mix the powder of the herbs in raw honey and let it set for a week. Then take a half-teaspoon morning and evening, or as needed to counter low energy and fatigue.

Aromatic Herbs, Oils and Incense

Aromatic herbs have powerful effects on the mind and prana, activating the higher brain centers. Other aromatic herbs help calm the mind and opening the heart. Such aromatic herbs can be used in the form of teas, essential oils, inhalants, nasya or as incense.[33]

Spicy aromatics like gingers, mints and sages are better at stimulating the mind and promoting insight and perception good for the yoga of knowledge or for Raja Yoga. They also help clear the head and sinuses and stimulate the flow of prana. They increase pranagni or the agni of the pranic sheath, which is good for pranayama.

Flower fragrances like jasmine and rose are better at opening the heart for devotion. Flower fragrances calm the outer mind and its emotional and sensory overloads, connecting us to a deeper level of feeling. They build ojas at a subtle level.

Spicy Aromatics: camphor, eucalyptus, peppermint, sage,

thyme, cinnamon, ginger, tea tree oil, wintergreen, tulsi

Sweet Flower Fragrances: *jasmine, rose, saffron, sandalwood, champak, iris, lotus, frangipani, honeysuckle*

Oil Massage and Yoga

In addition to herbs, we should not forget the value the external application of oils, particularly sesame oil, for counteracting rigidity of the joints and muscles and nourishing the deeper tissues of the body. Ayurvedic medicated oils, made by cooking special herbs in a sesame oil base, are especially important in this manner. They not only aid in yoga postures but treat diseases of the bones and nerve tissue. Oil massage can allow us to move into asanas that may have otherwise been impossible for us to do. It can help ground the prana so that our pranayama practices do not dry out the nervous system. Most of us can benefit from oily massage on a regular basis as part of our lifestyle regimens, particularly vata types.

Sesame oil has vata-counteracting properties. It aids in the flow of prana through the nadis and channels and increases ojas.

Coconut oil has pitta-counteracting properties. It is particularly useful to apply to the head, which tends to become overheated.

Mustard oil has kapha-counteracting properties. It is particularly useful to apply to the chest and lung region where kapha accumulates.

Ghee counters pitta and vata. It is mainly used for skin rashes of a dry or inflammatory nature which would be aggravated by other oils that are usually heating in nature.

Nasya and the Neti Pot

The neti pot is a small pot with a narrow spout used to pour water through the nostrils when the head is tilted back. A small amount of salt, an eighth of a teaspoon or so, is added to the lukewarm water. Herbs and oils can be also added to the neti pot as well for special or enhanced action. These include sesame oil and nervine herbs like brahmi, calamus, tulsi or ginger. One can also snuff the powder of various herbs like ginger or calamus to clear the sinuses. Or one can put ayurvedic oils, like medicated sesame oils, into the nostrils. The medicated oils are probably the best. They can cure many sinus allergies and also counter sinus headaches, dizziness, vertigo and brain fatigue. Yoga students should use ayurvedic nasya oils on a daily basis. They can do so after the neti pot or in place of it.

Pancha Karma

Pancha karma means the five purificatory practices. It consists of therapeutic enemas (basti), purgatives (virechana), emetics (vamana), nasal medications (nasya), and blood cleansing (rakta moksha) to eliminate excess doshas from the body. These follow a preparatory practice of oil massage (snehana) and steam therapy (svedana) to loosen up the toxins and bring them back to the digestive tract for their removal.

Purgatives increase apana (downward motion) to reduce pitta. Emetics stimulate udana (upward motion) to reduce kapha. Nasya opens the head to promote prana. Blood-cleansing stimulates the flow of blood through vyana to reduce pitta. Bastis or enemas calm apana in order to calm vata. In this way pancha karma works on all five pranas.

Pancha karma radically remove toxins not only from the physical body but also from the subtle body. It has a powerful cleansing and rejuvenating effect upon the bones, muscles and nerves, senses and mind. Therefore pancha karma is a helpful procedure for anyone on a yogic path, not only for asana but for pranayama and meditation. Pancha karma can be done as part of a detoxification program, to start a deeper level of practice, or as a regular measure to prevent the toxins from accumulating.[34]

14

Asana

Yoga Postures for Health and Awareness

From asana arises steadiness of body and mind,
freedom from disease and lightness of the limbs.

HATHA YOGA PRADIPIKA I.17

Yoga postures or asanas are one of the most important systems of physical culture ever invented. They reflect an amazing understanding of how the body works and, particularly, how to release tension at a deep level from the tissues, organs and joints.

Asanas keep the body in the best possible health. They provide specific positions and movements designed to strengthen and stretch the musculature to effectively move the body away from small pains and illnesses back to perfect and normal balance. They keep the spinal column subtle in order to create the optimal flow of energy through the nerves that enervate the organ and glandular systems. And, perhaps most importantly, they begin a systematic cleansing of the tissues preparing the body for more advanced yogic practices.

Asanas are a part of a sacred science that comprehends all aspects of consciousness. They are not only significant in themselves, but are a preparation for pranayama and meditation. They reflect not only a profound knowledge of the body but also of prana, mind and spirit, of which the body is only an external image or manifestation. In the present chapter we will explore the role of asana in yoga and Ayurveda.

Asana and the Greater System of Yoga

Asana is originally part of the deeper practices of yoga, but can also be done as exercise or as a therapy. Most people in the West perform asanas as exercise. This has become the meaning of yoga for them, which they associate with yoga postures. While asana can be a discipline in its own right, asana as exercise or as therapy should not be confused with the role of asana in classical yoga, which goes beyond this. Yoga should not be reduced to asana, which is only a fraction of the greater system.

Asana is mainly meant to help reduce rajas or the quality of turbulence that disturbs the mind (which is why a too active or assertive performance of asanas is counterproductive from a deeper yogic standpoint). Without proper asana to settle the prana, pranayama cannot proceed smoothly. Without proper asana to settle the senses, pratyahara or control of the senses is almost impossible. Without proper asana to settle the mind, concentration and meditation (dharana and dhyana) are very difficult. Those interested in the deeper stages of yoga should not neglect asana. They may benefit from a period of intense asana practice for a few years as part of physical purification. Then their body will not weigh them down as they seek to go deeper into the mind.

Yoga in the true sense of deep meditation usually occurs when the body is at rest in a sitting posture. When deep meditation happens, concern about asana fades away; the physical body and its position are forgotten. Many great yogis, we should note, were not great asana practitioners. Swami Vivekananda, for example, who first brought yoga to the West around the turn of the last century, was poor at asanas except for a few sitting postures. Similarly, many people who are good at asana may not be adept at deeper yogic meditational practices.

Of the different yoga paths, the yoga of knowledge (jnana yoga) places the least emphasis on asana. From its point of view, the cultivation of attention is the main thing. Similarly, the yoga of devotion (bhakti yoga) is not asana-oriented either. It emphasizes divine love and the attitude of the heart. Raja Yoga emphasizes meditation and makes asana important only in a preliminary sense. Hatha yoga is the main yoga that uses asana as a primary tool. Yet prana is more important in hatha yoga than asana practice.

Many great yogis learned their asanas from their own awakened prana, not from physical practice. In fact, prana is the original teacher of yoga postures, not mere human instruction. The true teacher of asana does so through awakening the prana of the student, not simply by teaching how to put the body into different poses. We should learn to use the power of prana to direct our asana practice from within, making it a creative process. When prana directs asana, its healing power is much greater. When prana is the focus of the asana practice and the movements (asanas) are placed on the flow of breath (prana) as pearls are placed on a string, then you have the practice of yoga as outlined by Patanjali in the *Yoga Sutras*.

Asana and Ayurveda

Ayurveda recommends asanas as its most important lifestyle recommendation for exercise. It also prescribes asanas as an important treatment measure for various diseases. Half of ayurvedic treatment is what goes into the body, which is mainly food. The other half is what the body does by way of expression, which is mainly exercise. Asana deals with this. Asana and food therefore are the two most important physical treatment measures in Ayurveda.

On the level of prana, herbs are the food and pranayama is the exercise. For these to work properly, the foundation of right posture and right diet in the physical body are necessary. A great variety of asanas is necessary to deal with the exercise and therapeutic requirements of different individual constitutions and their changing imbalances.

Asanas help treat all diseases but are rarely a complete treatment in themselves. Their action is mainly indirect, except in the case of musculoskeletal or structural problems. Asanas work to improve circulation to disease-affected areas in order to release toxins and improve the healing and growth of tissues. This catalyzes the body's healing processes on several levels.

Purpose of Asana

Asana is the main yogic tool for balancing the physical body. It consists of various static postures and physical movements performed to release tension, improve flexibility, maximize the flow of energy, and remove friction. The purpose of asana is to create a free flow of energy in order to help direct our attention within. But this flow of energy can also focused on the body to treat its ailments.

Our physical posture affects our health, vitality and awareness. The mind-body complex consists of various interrelated channels — from those which carry food to those which carry thoughts. These channels are held together on a physical level by the musculoskeletal system, the shape of which is determined by our posture.

Wrong posture creates various stresses, causing contractions that impair or block the proper flow through the channels. It inhibits the circulation of energy and nutrients while allowing toxins and waste materials to accumulate. Such blockages cause discomfort and reduce functioning, resulting in pain and disease. As mind and body are interconnected, physical blockages intertwine with mental and emotional blockages and hold various addictions, compulsions, and attachments.

Physical Body

The physical body (annamaya kosha) is centered in the digestive tract. If our posture is wrong then movement through the digestive tract gets obstructed. This disturbs or lowers the functioning of agni, the digestive fire, which in turn weakens or deranges digestion, leading to various ailments.

Tightness in the upper back and chest weakens the appetite, which is determined by the prana in the head and mouth. Tightness in the middle back and mid-abdomen weakens the digestive fire in the small intestine, which can become squashed by accumulated tension, causing malabsorption of food. Tightness or weakness in the lower back and abdomen constricts and weakens the colon. This creates gas and distention and upsets elimination, resulting in constipation or diarrhea and other problems of apana vayu.

Pranic Body

The pranic body (pranamaya kosha) works mainly through the respiratory and circulatory systems of the physical body. Oxygen, the physical counterpart of prana, is carried through the blood to energize all the tissues. If our posture is wrong then the lungs get impaired in their function. The breath becomes shallow and oxygen absorption is reduced. Mucus and stagnant air build up in the lungs, leading to congestion, infections and allergies. Resistance to air-borne pathogens is lowered along with poor immune function. Naturally, the posture of the upper and middle back strongly affects the lungs and circulation, particularly vyana vayu.

Wrong posture prevents the natural upward power of prana (udana vayu) through which we stand straight, feel happy and positive, and strive to grow and evolve in life. It causes apana, the downward energy, to increase along with feelings of heaviness, depression and lowering of energy.

Mind/Nervous System

The mental body works mainly through the head, brain and nervous system. If our posture is wrong then nerve impulses are disturbed. Tension in the neck reduces blood flow to the head and lowers mental energy. This contributes to headaches and sinus allergies, as well as other problems not only of the mind but of the pranic body.

The nervous system is closely connected with the skeletal system and, in ayurvedic thought, nerve tissue develops from bone tissue. Prana is held in the nerves and apana in the bones. The nervous system connects specifically to vata dosha, the biological air humor, which is the chief or guide of the other two doshas.

Wrong posture therefore aggravates vata primarily and disturbs the entire mind-body complex. Vata accumulates as cold and dryness in the bones and joints, leading either to stiffness and reduced movement or to tremors and disturbed movements. This tension gets transferred to the nerves, leading to insomnia, anxiety and emotional instability. The nervous system is governed by the spine, so all distortions of the spine will cause corresponding nerve tension and problems, mainly of a vata nature. By loosening the joints through yoga postures, the accumulated vata gets relieved, improving health and awareness on all levels. We can easily observe how fear and stress cause the body to tighten up. Such emotions get held in the bones and prevent our energy from moving freely.

Importance of Asana

Asana has tremendous therapeutic effects on body, prana and mind, on our physical structure, vital energy and creative intelligence. Unfortunately most of us today neglect our posture and do little to develop flexibility. Whatever exercise we do is usually of a strained or stressful type — aerobic exercises like running or weight lifting that cause further tension to accumulate and at best bring about only a one-sided development.

Anyone who works sitting at an office desk, particularly in the computer world of today, will tend to bad posture. Anyone who does a job that requires only one type of physical activity will have a posture that gets distorted in the direction of their work. Often our most comfortable lounging chairs also distort our posture during hours of resting or watching television.

Intellectual people, who are commonly vata in nature, neglect their bodies and hold them in stiff positions which makes flexibility decline. This can cause them to become hypersensitive owing to the accumulated vata in the bones. Traveling also aggravates vata for those who have jobs that require frequent flying or driving.

Yet even people who perform asanas on a daily basis may do so in a way that is not optimal. Asanas done forcefully or focused on the goal rather than on the process or journey — attempting to place the body in some ideal posture that is not natural to it — can result in tension or injury. Asana done without a cultivation of detachment, even if helpful on a physical level, can lead to an increased fixation on the body and rigidity of the mind and emotions.

Too much emphasis on asana also is not good. It can increase body consciousness and enhance the physical ego. If we really want to go into the full system of yoga, the time we spend doing asanas should not substitute for that spent in deeper practices of pranayama, mantra and meditation.

Asana and Age

Babies are naturally flexible and can do movements that adults, even those possessing great flexibility, are incapable of. Children are naturally physically active and athletic and like to play and run, exploring all the potentials of bodily movement. Childhood is the stage of life to begin asana practice to create a life-long foundation of right posture and flexibility.

Old age, beginning around the age of sixty-five, is the age of vata. Our bodily fluids gradually dry out along with declining vitality. The joints begin to stiffen, with loss of flexibility leading to arthritis. Asana is one of the best remedies for countering the effects of the aging process and for preventing vata from accumulating.

Movement-oriented asanas (*vinyasas*) are mainly for the young in whom the quality of rajas or action prevails. They need to develop their bodies and their minds are as yet immature. After the age of twenty-four, such movement asanas should gradually be replaced with a more internal form of asana practice emphasizing the development of the mind, particularly the study of spiritual teachings. After the age of forty-eight, one moves into the period when the inner mind develops as physical energies withdraw. During this time, one's meditation becomes more important than asana. After seventy-two, the mind develops yet further and physical energy begins to decline. This should be a period of deep meditation, yet it is necessary to continue asana to counter the aging process. It should be an integral part of our lifestyle regimen at any stage of life, even when it ceases to be our main concern in yoga.

Asana and Massage

Massage is an important tool for clearing toxins from the musculoskeletal system. Oil massage loosens the joints and nourishes the bones and nerves. Massage-related therapies like steam therapies, saunas and sweat lodges improve flexibility and remove toxins through the skin. After oil massage, asanas are easier to perform. Combined oil massage and steam therapies are a good aid to asana practice. A complete program of ayurvedic detoxification through pancha karma, using these procedures can take our asana practice to new level. However, massage can never substitute for asana. Regular asanas are essential to long term health. They are like giving oneself a massage and can be done more regularly and for longer periods of time.

Asana and Constitution

Asana is useful for all constitutions, though in different ways, and done right works to balance all the doshas. Everyone should practice at least half an hour a day of asana to prevent doshic excesses from developing. Asana is most needed by vata types, who are most prone to postural distortions. Kapha types, who tend to be sedentary and move slowly, benefit from more active forms of exercise, including more rajasic movement-oriented Asanas (vinyasas) or jumpings. Pitta types mainly need asanas to cool down their fiery and focused temperaments.

Which Asana to Do or How to Perform Asanas?

There are two main factors to consider in the practice of asana. The first is the manner and attitude with which the asanas are performed. The second is the particular asanas chosen. The first factor is the most significant. It is more important how we perform an asana than which particular asanas we do. The right asana done in the wrong way will not be helpful. On the other hand, an asana that may not be the best for a person's constitution, if done in the right manner and as part of a complete system of asana practice, can be beneficial. We may get the impression from ayurvedic books that the nature of the particular asana is the main thing, rather than how it is done. They list various asanas for different constitutions or diseases, as if one merely did the appropriate asana for the condition to be corrected. While specific asanas do relate to particular constitutions, they must be done correctly for their benefits to accrue.

Sometimes ayurvedic books recommend asanas that can be very difficult to do except for an advanced practitioner. The level of the student must not be forgotten in such instances. A beginner can get into a trouble trying to perform a difficult posture that is supposed to be good for their constitution but that they are not flexible enough to do properly. Our bodies need to be prepared for the new movements and different muscle loads we apply when doing asanas unfamiliar to us. For instance, the headstand, which has very valuable benefits, can be dangerous if done incorrectly or if the body is not properly prepared. Trying to force oneself into asanas is unwise.

Asana is not merely a simple matter of constitution. For example, the headstand is generally good for kapha, but a kapha person who is overweight and has a weak neck may be harmed by it. The particularities of individual bodily structure and organic condition cannot be forgotten. It is better to prescribe asanas according to the individual's condition and modify them according to ayurvedic considerations rather than to prescribe asana based upon ayurvedic constitution as the deciding factor.

In addition, individuals of one doshic constitution can suffer from diseases owing to another dosha. A vata person may have a kapha condition like a common cold, for example. Or a pitta person may come down with a vata condition, like insomnia, from too much traveling and overwork. In these instances, treatment aims at the dosha out of balance rather than at the person's constitutional type.

It is more important how we move into and maintain an asana than any technical perfection of form that we may be able to hold while in it. The main thing is to use the asana as a vehicle for directing the prana to the part of the body that one is seeking to benefit. Prana has the healing affect, not the asana by itself! For the prana to come into the posture requires linking the breath with the posture, which generally requires moving upon exhalation.

Moving into and adjusting an asana position while maintaining a strong focus on the breath creates a much deeper practice than simply focusing on body technique. This requires moving with prana, which means having one's attention focused on the free flow of energy, not on holding the body forcefully in a particular pose. Static asanas should arise through relaxation of effort, not through artificially holding a pose.[35]

The same asanas can be adjusted for different doshic types. Asanas done slowly, steadily and gently will generally reduce vata. Those done with coolness, diffusion of energy and relaxation will reduce pitta. Those done with quickness, heat and effort will reduce kapha. We can apply different forms of pranayama relative to asanas to either make them more heating or cooling, more building or reducing, further modifying their impact on the doshas. The application of asanas relative to different doshic types, therefore, requires adaptation and cannot be reduced to rigid rules.

Asanas are seldom done singly but as part of a sequence. During a sequence of asanas one can do various asanas for their benefits of exercising different muscles and joints, even if not all the asanas performed may be ideal for the constitutional type. The sequence as a whole should reduce the dosha. For example, pittas can do some heating asanas, even a headstand, but should do a practice dominated by and ending with cooling asanas. A complete practice will cover the full range of bodily motions and all main types of asanas, though each doshic type will require emphasizing some asanas more than others and doing them all in a manner that reduces their dosha.

Yoga Postures for Vata Constitution

Vata types are generally slight in built, with small bones and thin frames. They have a great deal of flexibility and agility when young but lack energy and stamina. They easily develop stiffness and rigidity as they age. Vata rules over the bones so vata types suffer most from arthritis, particularly after the age of fifty. They tend to be cold, with dry skin and cracking joints, along with poor circulation. Vata types are nervous and fearful. They commonly adapt a protective posture with raised shoulders and hunched back. They are also prone to scoliosis. Asana is a must for vata types. Without it they are unlikely to be healthy or have the stillness to meditate.

If we look at different asana practitioners, we will find that both the best and the worst will be mainly vata types. Vatas who maintain their flexibility through life-long physical activity will be the best (though they can suffer from too much flexibility, which causes instability if they over-exercise). It is important for vatas to remember to keep their spines flexible. Vata types who neglect their bodies and get too focused in their minds are likely to be the worst at asana practice. Vatas, being somewhat brittle and prone to excessive movement, are also most likely to be injured by wrong practice and too strong asanas. Vatas must approach asana carefully as they can easily hurt themselves.

Vatas need to perform asanas in a way that reduces vata, starting with the right mental attitude. They should never rush or hurry into asana practice. They should first put their minds in a calm space and place their emotions in a condition of rest. They should slow down and deepen their breath before beginning any postures. Vatas should warm up their bodies gradually, improving their circulation and loosening their joints. They should be aware of overexertion or of attempting postures before their bodies are ready. They should exercise to the point of a mild sweat only and make sure to have good fluid intake during the exercise period. A gentle attitude and gradually flowing movements are best for them.

Asana practice for vata types should emphasize the pelvic region and colon, the main sites of vata. They should aim at releasing tension from the hips, lumbar spine and sacroiliac joints. In general their asanas should restrict movement in order to counter vata's tendency to excess activity. Too much movement and stretching can cause them to overstretch their ligaments and lose strength. However, when vata leads to rigidity, then asana practice should work to increase movement and pranic flow into the stiffened areas, but in a gradual and steady manner.

Sitting postures are good for vata, particularly those that create strength and stillness in the lower abdomen like siddhasana (lotus pose) and vajrasana. These postures help develop calm, increase groundedness and control apana vayu.

Since vata tends to accumulate in the spine, making it stiff, vatas should focus on keeping the spinal column supple by practicing spinal bending in every direction. Spinal twists like matsyedrasana are excellent, removing vata from the nervous system. Yet twists are good only as long as the breath is full — when the breath is reduced even a little by the partial shutting down of one lung that can happen during twists, vata increases at a fast rate.

Forward bends afford immediate relief for excess vata, producing calm and stillness. They are excellent for releasing vata in the back where it builds up as stiffness and tension. They remove excess vata out of the body through the joints. But they cannot remove all vata unless combined with backbends.

Backbends are excellent for reducing vata but must be done gently and slowly to be effective. Vata commonly causes kyphosis and curvature of the shoulders. This stiffness, if attacked too aggressively, can cause pain or injury. Strong backbends are sympathetic stimulation — flight or fight action in the body's chemistry — and so have a 'spacing-out' effect. Backbends, if well grounded and done moderately, strengthen the vata's feelings of centeredness and have a warming effect, strengthening apana and the colon. Small backward bends, like cobra and locust, are the safest in this regard. More complete backbends can be done once proficiency in these is gained.

Standing postures that emphasize strength, stability and calm are very good for vata, particularly those that aim at developing stillness and balance like the tree pose (vrksasana). But vatas need to develop patience and concentration in order to appreciate them.

Vata people require gentle yoga procedures that do not exhaust them. They should only exert themselves moderately. They should follow any movement asanas with longer periods of sitting postures. To control vata they should practice pranayama and meditation in those postures.

After asana practice, vatas should make sure to rest and relax through the practice of the corpse pose. They should not end their practice abruptly or hurry off into any disturbing activity. Vatas should come away from asana practice feeling stable, warmed and calm, with tension released from the lower abdomen. Their minds should feel peaceful and emotions steady and grounded, with both space and energy for meditation.

Yoga Postures for Pitta Constitution

Pitta types have medium or average builds. They are neither too tall nor too short in height, neither too heavy nor too thin in weight. They usually possess a good musculature and flexibility owing to their good circulation and the oily quality of pitta that lubricates the joints. When they dedicate themselves to asana practice, pittas become quite good at it. Still they may lack the ability of long-boned vata types to do certain postures. They can also make their joints too loose from excessive practice, which can create problems just as significant as too much stiffness in the joints.

Psychologically, pittas are aggressive and like to excel and shine at what they do. They may take their high achievement mentality into asana practice where it is not appropriate. This can make them good at the technical side of asana but in the process they can lose the spiritual effect of practice, which depends upon peace of mind. Pitta people are often overly ambitious, irritable or driven. Yoga postures should be used to cool them down both on the physical and emotional levels. This helps them direct their intelligence within, where they can use it to understand themselves.

Pittas should perform asanas in a way that is cooling, nurturing, expansive and relaxing. This requires relaxing breaths and quiet sitting between strong asanas to release any stress that is developing. They should be careful not to turn their practice into a strong workout in which additional heat is generated in the body or in which too much sweating occurs. They should avoid overheating the blood or bringing too much heat to the head. This does not mean that they cannot do any strong practice but that they should make sure to compensate for any heat created by ending with cooling postures and cooling pranayama.

According to the yogic understanding of the body, the solar principle is centered around the navel, the place of the digestive fire that brings heat to the body. The lunar principle is located in the region of the soft palate, where salivary secretions constantly take place that have a cooling and moistening effect. The upward moving heat of the sun in the navel works to reduce the activity of the moon in the soft palate. Putting the body regularly into the shoulder stand or plow pose protects the lunar principle from the depleting heat of the solar principle and creates coolness. Such postures help reverse the positions of the sun and the moon in the body, bringing balance. This is naturally beneficial for pittas. Spinal twists, like Matyendrasana, are also very good for protecting the lunar principle without reducing agni or the power of digestion

Pitta people are benefited by postures that aim at releasing tension from the mid-abdomen, the small intestine and liver, where pitta accumulates. Such are the bow pose, cobra pose, boat pose, and fish pose. These postures allow excess pitta to be eliminated from the body, particularly to flow downward through the digestive tract. Headstands create pitta and should not be done unless one knows how to balance out the heat that they create.

Forward bends are generally good for pitta because they bring more energy to the mid-abdomen and have a cooling and grounding effect if done in a gentle manner. Backbends tend to be heating and so should be done only with moderation and followed by cooling postures. Seated twists help clear the liver, detoxifying pitta. Pittas should come away from asana practice feeling cool, content and calm, with tension released from the mid-abdomen. Their minds should be clear and relaxed, their emotions at rest, with no feelings of competitiveness or irritation. Their awareness should be in a meditative mood, slightly diffused and not overly sharp.

Yoga Postures for Kapha Constitution

Kapha types possess stocky builds and hold weight easily. They are generally shorter than average in height but sometimes are tall. Their frame, however, is always bulky with short bones and generally poor flexibility. For this reason kaphas should not try to force themselves into positions like the lotus pose, which are not appropriate for the type of joints that they have, or they can get hurt. Kapha people should not imagine themselves as tall skinny yogis. That is not their body type and it is not possible for them to maintain that build, even if they should be able to achieve it temporarily.

Kapha women may be thin when young but easily gain weight when they get older, particularly after childbirth. This often disturbs them and causes them to pursue weight loss programs, including through yoga postures, at which they are seldom successful. They must learn to accept their builds and not try to force their bodies into a shape that is unnatural to them. However, kaphas must strive to avoid overweight, which is to hold a moderate body weight, not to try to starve themselves.

Overweight in kapha types results in accumulation of fat, particularly in the stomach and thighs. This shifts the center of gravity downward, causing stooped shoulders and other postural problems. Kapha also creates mucus in the region of the chest which then moves to different sites in the body, particularly downward. It inhibits movement through the channels by its heavy and damp quality. It increases fat along the joints and the surface of the body. It builds up in the joints as an excessive synovial fluid. Such excess kapha causes swollen glands, benign cysts, and bone spurs. Many kaphas develop arthritis as a complication of such overweight or poor circulation.

Kapha types tend to be sedentary and seldom are physically active unless stimulated or prodded to do so, particularly after childhood. More active exercise is required for them, stimulating their metabolism and increasing circulation. However, kaphas should increase their exercise in a slow and incremental manner, particularly if they are severely overweight. As kaphas are prone to heart disease and high cholesterol, care must be taken not to overstrain their hearts in any exercise program.

Kapha is like a frozen river. Its movement is inhibited by cold. As heat is applied through exercise and deep breathing, the ice begins to melt. It then breaks off in chunks and flows downstream. Such kapha, as it moves out of areas of stagnation, can cause problems elsewhere if it is pushed out too forcefully.

Kaphas benefit by exercise that causes them to sweat, even profusely, and pushes them beyond what they think is the limit of their exertion (unless they are severely overweight, in which case caution is required). Generally kaphas should be made to do stronger exercise than they like and must be taught to challenge themselves.

Sitting asanas, like any condition of reduced movement, causes kapha to increase. Kaphas easily feel tired or fall into daydreaming when holding seated postures. To benefit by sitting postures, which is necessary for meditation, kaphas must practice pranayama of a warming nature.

Vinyasas, like the sun salutation with its constant activity, are stimulating to the kapha constitution. Standing postures in general are good for them, particularly as combined with movement and stretching. Virabhadrasana and its variations are good, particularly aimed at opening the chest, the place in the body where kapha accumulates. Backward bends are generally good for kaphas because they open the chest and increase circulation to the head, where mucus easily builds up for them, blocking the senses and dulling the mind. Forward bends, which tend to contract the chest, are not as good for them except when they are caught up in emotional distress and seek some short term calming influence.

Kapha people usually have slow digestion and low metabolism. To stimulate the digestive capacity, procedures having an action on the navel region (where agni is situated) are very useful (like *nauli*). The bow pose is the one of most beneficial of yoga postures for them because of this. To counter kapha congestion or stagnation, the right yoga postures combined with pranayama are excellent. This brings more circulation to both body and mind so that they can change their lives in a positive direction. The plow pose is one of the best for opening the lungs for kapha.

Kaphas should come away from asana practice feeling invigorated, warm and light, with their circulation energized, their chest and lungs open. Their mind and senses should be sharp and clear, with emotional heaviness released and forgotten.

Good Asanas for the Doshic Types

The following are generally good postures for the different doshic types, but again remember that the particularities of an individual's body structure and organic condition are more important than the doshic type in asana practice.

Vata

Key Words for Practice
• Calm, slow, steady, grounding, strengthening and consistent

Asanas

• Sitting poses like Lotus Pose (Siddhasana), Diamond Pose (Vajrasana), Lion Pose, Virasana.
• Sun Salutation done slowly and consciously.
• Standing poses like the Vrksasana (Tree Pose), Trikonasana

(Triangle), Virabhadrasana (Warrior Poses), Parighasana (Gate Pose) and all standing forward bends.

- Inverted poses like Headstand, Viparitakarani (a relaxing inversion).

- Cobras and Locusts (simple back bending), done consciously and carefully.

- Forward bends of all types, especially Janu Sirsasana (head-knee forward bend) and Paschimottanansana (full forward bend).

- Fetal position, Kurmasana (Tortoise), Parivrtta Janu Sirsasana (turning head-knee), Navasana (Boat Pose), Yoga Mudra (Yogic Seal).

- Spinal twists, especially lying twists, Bharadvajasana II (Sage Twist), Pasasana (Noose twist).

- Corpse pose: vatas need to do a long and comfortable relaxation of at least 20 minutes.

Pitta

Key Words for Practice

- Cooling, relaxing, surrendering, forgiving, gentle, diffusive

Asanas

- Sitting postures in general, except Lion Pose.

- Moon salutation (Chandra Namaskar).

- Standing poses, especially hips open poses like the Tree Pose, Trikonasana (Triangle Pose), and Ardha Chandrasana (Half Moon).

- Legs open standing forward bends like Prasarita Padottanasana I (extended spread legs).

- Shoulder stand, Viparitikarani, Boat Pose, Fish Pose, Cobra

Pose, Bow Pose, Fetal Pose .

- All sitting forward bends, especially Upavistha Konasana, and Kurmasana (Tortoise), Paschimottanasana.
- Twists like Ardha Matsyendrasana II and Maricyasana.
- Yoga Mudra (Yogic Seal), Corpse Pose.

Kapha

Key Words for Practice

- Stimulating, moving, warming, lightening, energizing, releasing

Asanas

- Lion pose or sitting poses with pranayama.
- Sun salutation, strong vinyasas or 'jumpings.'
- Virabhadrasana, Utthita Hasta Padangusthasana (extended hand toe), Urdhva Prasarita Ekapadasana (extended foot above), Ardha Chandrasana (Half Moon),
- Downward Dog (Adho Mukha Svanasana), Upward Dog (Urdhva Mukha Svanasana).
- Full inverted balancing poses like handstand (Adho Mukha Vrksasana), Pinca Mayurasana (Peacock Feather pose).
- Headstand and shoulder stand with variations.
- Plow pose, all backbends like Upward Bow Pose, Camel Pose (Ustrasana), and Locust Pose, Jathara Parivartanasana (Alligator Twist) or Maricyasana followed by a short Savasana.

Description of Particular Asanas

The following descriptions are intended mainly for those who already know the asanas in order to help them to orient their practice in an ayurvedic light. For those unfamiliar with the asanas, please consult yoga books and teachers for a more complete description of how to do them. When in doubt, do not attempt any movements that may cause strain or stress. The ayurvedic indications for the asanas are only general. As much depends upon the manner and sequence in which the asana is performed as the nature of the asana itself. In some instances there are several variations on the posture, not all of which will be equally good for each individual. I have tried to avoid listing postures that are hard to do or advanced.

I. SITTING POSES

Sitting postures are the most important in yoga. All other postures are to bring us to the point of being able to hold sitting poses. Classical yoga, with its prime aim of meditation, emphasizes four sitting asanas: lotus pose, siddhasana, vajrasana, and lion pose. These are good for pranayama and meditation. Any comfortable sitting posture on a chair or on the floor can be used in place of these.

STAFF POSE (Dandasana)

Dandasana is the basic sitting pose. All of the sitting poses begin and end in dandasana. Sit on the floor, mat, or carpet with the legs stretched out straight in front. Pull the flesh of the buttocks back on each side so that you may sit directly on the sitting bones. Inhale and extend through the straight legs and out through the heels, moving the balls of the feet toward the face. Place the hands on the floor beside the back of the hips (fingers facing forward) and push down to lift the chest up and forward. The spine is straight with the back lifting upward on each exhalation. The hands remain in the same place, but now take the weight off the hands and keep lifting the torso up and extending the legs out. Maintain this posture, breathing comfortably.

The staff pose is especially good for calming vata and pitta, and also reduces kapha. It helps strengthen udana in particular.

EASY POSTURE (Sukhasana)

Sit in dandasana with the legs stretched out in front. Then bend the legs and cross the right shin over the left, folding the feet under the legs. In this easy 'crossed-legs' position, keep your spine erect. Rest your hands (separated) on your knees. Or cup the left hand (palms up) in the right hand, thumbs touching, and rest them on your lap.

This posture is for those who cannot do more difficult seated postures. It has similar benefits for facilitating pranayama and meditation.

LOTUS POSTURE (Padmasana)

Sit in sukhasana. With both hands, lift the right foot and ankle and gently place them on top of the left thigh with the right heel near the left groin. Then take the left foot and ankle and lift them over the right leg, gently placing them on the right thigh. The soles of the feet are turned upward as the tops of the feet rest on the thighs. Keep the spine erect and close the eyes. Place the palm of the left hand on the palm of the right hand, keeping the hands together between the heels.

The lotus pose regulates vata, controls apana vayu and allows for the prana to move into the sushumna. It is the best posture for pranayama and pratyahara, and excellent for meditation.

SIDDHASANA

Sit on a mat with legs stretched out. Bend the right knee and place the heel of the right foot under the perineum. Now bend the left leg, placing the left heel on top of the right heel and against the pubic bone. Keep the head, neck and back straight. Fix the gaze at the third eye. With the tops of the hands on the knees, make jnana mudra (sign of knowledge) by touching the thumb with the index finger. Keep the other three fingers straight, palms facing upward.

Siddhasana is perhaps the best posture for concentration and meditation and promotes spiritual knowledge. It calms vata, controls apana and keeps prana moving upward. It does not aggravate the other doshas.

DIAMOND POSE (Vajrasana)

Sit down on bent knees so that the calves touch the thighs. Place both heels close to each other and then sit on the heels. Place the palms over the respective knees. Keep the body straight and look straight forward.

Diamond pose is excellent posture for pranayama, particularly of the heating type like right nostril breathing, bhastrika, and kapalabhati. It helps awaken prana and kundalini and is excellent for stimulating pranagni.

LION POSE (Simhasana)

Sit down placing the left foot beneath the right hip and the right foot beneath the left. Spread the fingers like the claws of a lion and place them on the knees. Draw the stomach inward and spread the chest forward. Open the mouth wide and stick out the tongue as much as possible. With open eyes gaze at the third eye.

Lion pose increases agni and pitta on all levels, energizing the head, eyes, throat and digestive system. It reduces kapha and vata, countering cold and low energy.

II. STANDING POSES

MOUNTAIN POSE (Tadasana)

Tadasana is the basic standing posture. It is the position that each standing pose begins from and returns to when completed. Stand upright with feet hip distance apart and parallel. Be aware of both feet evenly contacting the floor and balance the weight evenly on the balls and heels of the feet (toes remain relaxed). Strengthen the muscles in the legs and pull the knees up. Lift the hips up away from the legs. Continue the lift by stretching the spine upward from the tailbone through the top of the head. The shoulders are relaxed back and down. The arms and hands hang relaxed at the sides.

Tadasana is a grounding pose that balances all doshas if performed in the right manner. The right posture for standing sets the basic tone of our bodily posture, particularly for movement.

TRIANGLE POSE (Trikonasana)

Stand in tadasana. Spread the feet 3-4 feet apart. Turn the right foot, knee and leg 90 degrees to the right. Turn the left foot in slightly, keeping the left leg straight. Stand with the weight on the outsides of the feet, arches lifting. Breathe in and raise the arms out to the sides to shoulder level. Exhale and bend the entire torso to the right, keeping the spine straight and the shoulders vertically over the right leg. The chest opens toward the ceiling as the spine continues to lengthen out to the right. Breathe fully holding the position. Inhale to lift the body back to standing and, with an exhalation, return back to tadasana. Repeat to the left side.

Trikonasana is good for all doshas, particularly for vata and vyana.

WARRIOR II (Virabhadrasana)

Stand in tadasana. Spread the feet approximately 5 feet apart. Breathe in and raise the arms out to the sides and up to shoulder level. Exhale and turn the right foot, knee, and leg 90 degrees to the right. Turn the left foot in slightly by moving the left heel out. Stand with the weight on the outsides of the feet, arches lifting. As you exhale, bend the right knee to 90 degrees,

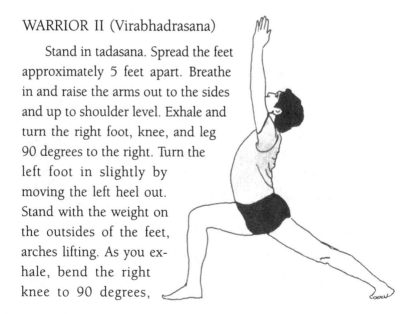

shin vertical to the floor with the hips facing forward (as much as possible while keeping the right knee over the right heel). Keep the left leg and knee very straight both when coming down into the pose and in maintaining it. The lower back lengthens down as the chest opens forward and up. Stretch out through the arms and hands while keeping the shoulders down away from the ears. Maintain this position while breathing comfortably and evenly. On an exhale, return to tadasana. Repeat to the other side.

Virabhadrasana opens the chest and lungs. It increases pranagni and vyana and reduces kapha. It is grounding and stabilizing to vata.

EXTENDED ANGLE POSE (Parsvakonasana)

Stand in tadasana. Spread the feet about 5 feet apart. Breathe in and raise and stretch

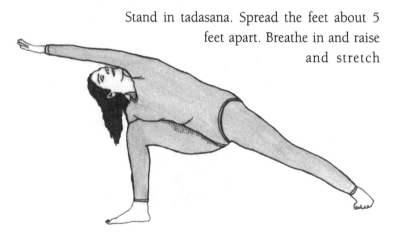

the arms sideways to shoulder level. Exhale and turn the right foot 90 degrees to the right. Turn the left foot in slightly by moving the left heel out. Stand with the weight on the outsides of the feet, arches lifting. As you exhale, bend the right knee to ninety degrees and come into virabhadrasana II. Keep the left leg and knee very straight. Lengthen and bend the torso sideways down to the right and put the right hand on the floor behind the right foot. The right side of the torso is in line with the right thigh and the chest revolves toward the ceiling. Turn the head and look up in front of the outstretched left arm that is alongside the left ear. Breathe normally as you maintain this pose, then inhale and come back to virabhadrasana II. Exhale and move back to tadasana. Repeat on the other side.

A grounding posture, parsvakonasana mainly reduces vata and kapha.

III. INVERTED POSES

DOWNWARD FACING DOG (Adho Mukha Svanasa)

Begin on the hands and knees with the hands under the shoulders and the knees hip distance apart under the hips. Inhale and keep the arms straight. Exhale, push the buttocks up toward the ceiling, straightening the legs. Standing on the balls of the feet (the heels up) drop your head so that you look towards your feet. From the wrists to the tailbone, the body is in a straight line. With the tailbone held up, keep lengthening the arms and torso as you let the heels come down toward the floor. Breathe comfortably as you maintain this posture. Then bend the knees, sit back on the heels, put the head on the floor and rest in fetal pose.

Dog pose is especially energizing for kapha and grounding for vata. It helps balance all the doshas.

SUPPORTED SHOULDER STAND (Salamba Sarvangasana)

Lay flat on your back. Bend your knees and bring your legs up to your chest and swing them over your head until you have raised your trunk and legs to vertical, while bending at the neck with your shoulders and arms supporting you on the ground. Rest your elbows on the ground firmly and support the back with both palms. The whole body weight should rest on your shoulders and arms (you may need to use folded wool blankets under the torso and shoulders with the head and neck on the floor to soften the strain on the neck and head). Keep the body still and hold the posture breathing comfortably. To come down, bend the knees and, using the arms for support on the floor behind you, slowly unroll the spine back to the ground until the back and feet rest on the floor.

The shoulder stand regulates udana vayu and kapha in the region of the chest. It counters high pitta (unless we hold the posture too long) and reverses apana vayu. It is a good blood purifier and nourishes the brain, throat and lungs. Good for hypothyroidism, relieves headaches and counters constipation.

RESTORATIVE INVERSION (Viparitakarani)

Place a bolster or an 8-12 inch pile of well-folded blankets against a wall. Sit sideways at the edge of the blankets with one sitting bone on the blankets and one on the wall. With the hands on the floor for support, bend and then swing the legs up the wall as you turn onto your back to lie on the floor and blankets. The legs are straight up the wall. Keep the sitting bones against the wall and the hips and low back on the blankets. The shoulders, neck, and head are on the floor and the arms are relaxed over the head on the floor. Hold the position comfortably for some time, then bend the knees and gently roll over to the side and off the blankets.

Viparitakarani is a relaxing pose that keeps the chest open and the breathing relaxed as the blood moves down into the head and shoulders. Reduces excess tension in the brain and mind. Excellent for headaches, migraines and sinus conditions, and improving circulation to the head. Can be used to balance all the doshas.

IV. BACKBENDS

EASY COBRA POSE (Bhujangasana)

Lay face down on the mat. Keep the legs together, forehead touching the ground, and the soles of the feet facing up. The palms are flat on the ground under the shoulders, elbows bent and close to the sides. First raise the head slowly, moving the face up, then the head and then the neck, shoulders, and sternum. Allow the upper portion of the body to follow as the back of the head continues to lift upward (chin does not extend forward). During this time no weight should be placed on the hands as initially the back muscles should be strengthened. After maintaining this position for some time, extend the chest forward to unroll the spine back to the lying-down position.

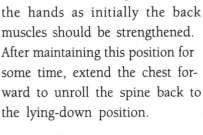

The cobra pose harmonizes pitta and regulates samana vayu, stimulating agni. It calms vata in the colon and improves circulation in the digestive region. It also stimulates kundalini, whose energy is like a cobra.

FISH POSE (Matsyasana)

From lying on the back, raise the torso up onto the forearms, elbows, and hands. The elbows are beside the torso and under the shoulders, fingertips are under the hips. Arch the upper back and lean backward, shifting the body weight back and the head toward the floor. Gently place the upper back of the head on the floor, still supporting the weight with the arms and hands. Inhale and continue arching the back and neck. As you gain strength in the back and shoulders, you may want to ease away some of the support of the arms and slowly move them down under your hips. Maintain comfortably in this arched back position for a few moments, then ease the arms out from under you and relax down to the lying position.

The fish pose increases agni and helps move pitta out of the digestive system and liver. It is also good for the throat and lungs.

V. FORWARD BENDS

SEATED ANGLE (Upavistha Konasana)

Sit in dandasana with the legs stretched out straight in front. Inhale and open the legs as wide apart as possible. Exhale, extend out through the heels, straightening the legs and bringing the balls of the feet back toward the face. The kneecaps face the ceiling and do not roll in or out. Use the fingertips on the floor behind the hips to push up to straighten the spine. Keep the spine (including the neck) straight, extending up through

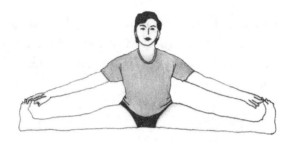

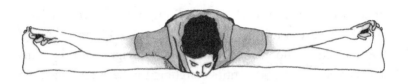

the top of the head as you move forward bringing the torso toward the floor. Breathe comfortably and maintain the posture. Then inhale as you move back to dandasana.

The seated angle reduces pitta and vata, increasing calm and steadiness.

FULL FORWARD BEND (Paschimotanasana)

Sit in dandasana with the spine erect and the legs and heels extended. Inhale and stretch the arms up to the ceiling, drawing the spine upward. Hold the length of the spine as you exhale and move the low abdomen forward toward the thighs. Keeping the shoulders back and the chest open, continue to breathe and move the trunk slowly forward until you can hold onto the legs or feet. As you inhale, strengthen the legs and push out through the heels. As you exhale, lengthen the spine and move further forward until your trunk is stretched along the thighs (with the spine and neck still straight) and your face moves to your shins. Hold this posture working with the breath for a minute or two and then return to dandasana.

Paschimotanasana regulates apana vayu, strengthens digestion, and is cooling to the head. Also it can be used to pull the chest forward and reduce kapha. As with most forward bends, it soothes vata imbalance and is excellent for reducing pitta.

VI. TWISTS

ALLIGATOR TWISTS (Jathara Parivartanasana)

There are 4 positions for this easy, comfortable twist. The instructions are the same for each position with the exception of the foot and leg position. For each position begin by lying on the back.

Position #1: Keep the legs and feet together and straight (center). Lie on the back. Stretch the arms out sideways until they are at right angles to the body. Inhale, pushing through the heels and straightening the legs. Exhale, turning the hips and legs to the right as you let the head move to the left. Remain in this position with the spine rotated for a few moments, then inhale and move back to center. Exhale and rotate the hips to the left side, letting the head turn to the right. Breathe as you hold the position for a few moments and then return to center with the inhalation.

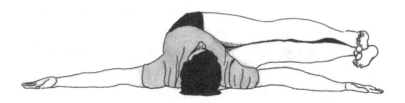

Position #2: One leg is bent with its foot placed on the knee of the straight other leg. Follow the instruction for breathing and turning as written in Position #1.

Position #3: Both knees are bent and brought to the chest to begin. Follow the instruction for breathing and turning as written in Position #1.

Position #4: The completed pose, both legs are straight and in the air perpendicular to the torso. Follow the instruction for breathing and turning as written in Position #1.

This simple twisting movement is very beneficial for improving circulation to the spine and nadis, especially for vyana, vata and pitta.

FULL SPINAL TWIST (Ardha Matsyendrasana)

Sit in dandasana. Bend the left leg in and place the foot underneath the buttocks. Place a folded blanket under the foot for comfort. With the top of the left foot down and at a right angle to the ankle, sit on the left heel so that the right sitting bone is directly on the arch of the foot (Note reflexology for the foot working on the spine).

The left knee faces forward. Now take the right foot over the left knee to the floor on the outside of it. The right knee is facing the ceiling. Press the floor with the fingertips and elongate the spine upward. Sitting into the left foot, slowly turn to the right (beginning the rotation from the base of the spine). Place the left arm on the outside of the right knee, with the hand and

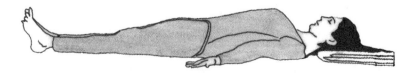

forearm vertical. (Right fingertips are still on the floor assisting with lift and balance) With the ribs lifted turn the abdomen. The pose is completed by bringing the back of the left armpit in contact with the right knee and moving the back of the left arm around to encircle the right knee, clasping the right wrist with the right arm behind you. It is most important that the breath should remain full and steady at all times in twisting poses. Remain in the pose for 20-40 seconds, then on an exhalation release the arms and legs and repeat to other side.

This twist strengthens the spine, counters scoliosis, improves digestion, and reduces vata. It helps detoxify the liver, removing heat from the small intestine, reducing pitta.

THE FINAL POSE FOR EVERY ASANA PRACTICE

CORPSE POSE (Savasana)

Lay down comfortably on the back with the legs stretched long and slightly apart. Make sure to keep the body warm. Pull the shoulders down and tuck them under you as you lengthen the arms along the floor, palms up. Arms and hands are kept slightly away from the torso. Lengthen the neck and head. Inhale deeply. Exhale and allow the whole body to let go and comfortably relax. Systematically release all tension held in each part of the body. Then let go of the mind by focusing on the breath and its movement through the body. Completely relax in this way for 20 minutes.

Savasana is considered to be the most important asana and always follows and completes any asana practice. It helps relieve accumulated vata or stress, particularly at the end of asana practice, and cools down pitta as well.

15

Methods of Pranayama

*The sacred syllable Om, the fire of Prana,
the Supreme Self, surrounded by the five Pranas;
it is the ruler of the entire universe.*

BRIHADYOGI YAJNAVALKYA SMRITI, IX.10

We are all in pursuit of prana as our main activity in life, whether we are aware of it or not. Human enjoyment proceeds through the power of prana alone. The pleasure that we feel in eating, in sex, in watching a movie, in running, skiing, jumping or any activity of the sensory and motor organs are all due to prana alone. However, because we are not in control of our prana, we can only produce pranic enjoyments according to external factors that remain limited and ultimately exhaust us.

Yoga teaches us how to master prana and unfold its deeper powers. The yogi learns to ride the waves of prana so that he can experience the bliss of prana in his own consciousness. He can take his mind into a state of great speed (prana), infinite expansion (vyana), unlimited ascension (udana), immutable calm (samana) or unbreakable endurance (apana). Once we learn to master prana we no longer require external forms of enjoyment. We gain power over the mind and senses. This same pranic force can be used to heal body and mind. A true ayurvedic doctor is a pranic healer who knows how to direct prana at will for the benefit of the patient, as well as how to use food, herbs and other healing substances as vehicles for prana.

According to the *Vedas*, the prana within the human body corresponds to the sun in the external world.[36] Just as the sun revolves around the sky, so prana revolves through the channel systems of the body and mind. Just as the sun measures time externally, so prana controls it internally. Therefore, the key to the movement of our lives and to taking us beyond the limit of time lies in our ability to control our prana. Just as learning to harness solar energy can transform the external world, so the development of pranic energy is the key to internal transformation.

Pranayama is one of the most central yoga practices, marking the fourth of the eight limbs of classical yoga. It is the prop on which the entire system of yoga rests. Prana purifies and energizes body and mind for higher meditational practices, without which we lack the energy to pursue them properly. We have already discussed the subject of prana and its five subtypes, and the three vital essences of prana, tejas and ojas. In this chapter we will examine specific pranayama practices, including for the five pranas.

Please note: Pranayama, particularly stronger types, should be learned from a teacher. The information presented here is not meant to substitute for personal instruction.

Prana means the vital force and *ayama* means expansion. Therefore pranayama means "expansion of the vital force." However, some people define pranayama as "retention of the breath." While retention of the breath, if done correctly, is probably the most powerful method to expand the vital force, it is not the only one. If done incorrectly, it can constrict the vital force and aggravate many diseases, just as failing to breathe causes us to faint. Through pranayama one slows down and extends the breath so that the inner prana or higher life-force can manifest.

This aids in slowing down and calming the mind, facilitating meditation.

Pranayama is an integral part of ayurvedic treatment methods and lifestyle regimens. It is most effective in treating diseases of the respiratory, circulatory and nervous systems, whose function depends upon the right flow of prana, yet it is excellent for all conditions of debility, low energy, chronic fatigue, weak immunity, and convalescence. It is probably the most important single action that we can do to improve our health. Life without pranayama is life without real prana.

Pranayama not only exercises the lungs but all the organs in the body through the internal massage action of inhalation and exhalation. This massaging action improves circulation to the organs and dispels toxins, bringing the doshas to the digestive tract for elimination. It sets up a deep and powerful organic rhythm to sustain not only health and strength but calmness of mind.

Pranayama is an important tool for treating psychological and emotional disorders. It is excellent to counter depression, release grief and attachment, and reduce stress and tension. It is much more effective in raising our spirits than any stimulant or drug. Pranayama enhances the power of tonic herbal therapies to improve vitality, like ginseng, ashwagandha or shatavari.

Working on Prana

There are many ways to work on prana. Proper nutrition increases prana on a physical level. This also requires proper elimination. According to Ayurveda, the prana from food is absorbed in the large intestine, particularly in the upper two-thirds, which is not simply an organ of elimination. Apana vayu, which resides in this organ, is the most important prana for physical health, insuring that no toxins can build up in the body. Laxative herbs, particularly the compound triphala, aid in the right absorption of prana from the food, helping to ground prana in the physical body and cut off the root of physical disease.

The *Vedas* say that mortals eat food with apana (the vital force in the lower abdomen), while the gods eat food with prana (the vital force in the head).[37] The mortals are the physical tissues; the immortals are the senses that imbibe nourishment directly through the sense openings in the head. While right food sustains apana, right impressions are required to feed prana. For this contact with nature, rituals and visualizations are important, as well as sensory therapies involving colors, sounds or aromas. As we grow spiritually we must learn to take in more prana to feed the gods or spiritual powers within us. We need to control apana, particularly the sexual urge, so that we don't lost our vital energy downward.

Mantras, particularly single syllable or bija mantras like OM or HRIM, create vibrations (nada) that direct pranic energy in the entire mental field, including the subconscious. Meditation itself, creating space in the mind, generates prana in the mind. When the mind is brought into a silent and receptive state, like the expanse of the sky, a new prana comes into being within it that heals and integrates our awareness. Wherever space and stillness is created, prana or energy must follow. However, the main method for working on prana and pranamaya kosha is pranayama or yogic breathing exercises.

Balancing Prana and Apana

Apana, which is aligned with the force of gravity, moves downward resulting in disease, aging, death and the diminution of consciousness. Prana, which is aligned with the air and space elements, disperses upward through the mind and senses. This leads to loss of mind-body coordination and devitalization.

Uniting these two prime pranas results in strengthening our energy along with awakening our higher faculties. Yogic practices work to raise apana up to unite with prana and draw prana down to unite with apana, which occurs in the region of the navel — the pranic center in the body.

Pranayama and Pranagni

Pranayama develops pranagni or the agni of prana, which is responsible for the digestion of prana in the body. Pranagni develops primarily through correct retention of the breath that follows deep inhalation. Inhaled oxygen is food for pranagni; exhaled carbon dioxide is its waste material. Just as fasting purifies the physical body, so breath retention purifies the subtle body. Pranagni creates a special form of sweating that eliminates the toxins that block the various nadis.

The navel, in which all the pranas unite, is also the center of pranagni in the physical body, the agni of prana, which gets enkindled through the union of prana and apana. The navel is the highest of the three lower chakras that are all interconnected. Pranagni gives rise to the kundalini force that awakens these chakras and rises upward, carrying both prana and apana with it.

Prana, Tejas and Ojas

To practice pranayama rightly we must first build ojas, the vital essence of kapha. Ojas serves as the fluid that holds prana, without which the prana will disperse. It is the wire through which the pranic current can flow. To practice pranayama without developing ojas can cause vata disorders, anxiety, insomnia and ungroundedness. Without the proper ojas to support it, pranayama will dry out the nervous system.

Conversely, prana energizes and purifies ojas. The additional prana taken in through pranayama dries and evaporates ojas in order to bring it to the higher head centers. If we are accumulating ojas, particularly through sexual abstinence, we should practice pranayama to convert it. Otherwise it will accumulate, become heavy, and by a gravitational force disperse its energy downward.

Prana also energizes tejas, like wind does a fire. This gives us fiery vital energy, courage and fearlessness. If we do not develop the prana then the energy of tejas also cannot endure. Pranayama aids in developing tejas, which is the expression of pranagni, the fire of prana. Note the chapter on prana, tejas and ojas.

Pranayama and the Five Pranas

While pranayama is usually defined as balancing prana and apana, eventually all five pranas must be considered. Vyana and samana both relate to retention. Samana is the initial stage of retention in which the air is consolidated in the lungs, with oxygen absorbed through the lung tissue. Vyana is the second stage of retention in which the absorbed oxygen is taken into the blood and carried to the rest of the body.

Udana and apana both relate to exhalation. Udana is the first stage of exhalation that creates positive energy and effort, which allows for speech. Apana is the second stage of exhalation that pushes out the waste air and carbon dioxide. Through pranayama we can balance and regulate all five pranas.

THE FIVE PRANAS AND THE BREATH

Prana — Inhalation
Samana — Retention/Contraction
Vyana — Retention/Expansion
Udana — Exhalation/Expression
Apana — Exhalation/Elimination

Pranayama and the Doshas

Pranayama treats all the doshas. The right practice of pranayama normalizes vata, the master dosha and expression of prana. Pranayama is one of the main practices for reducing kapha, which has a tendency to stagnation and the production of mucus. It helps reduce kapha in both the head and lungs. In addition, special cooling pranayamas counter pitta and remove heat. The use of prana for healing is an important aspect of Ayurveda that should never be overlooked in treatment.

Inhalation, like eating, relates to kapha and has a building effect. Retention, like digestion, relates to pitta and has a transforming effect. Exhalation, like elimination, relates to vata and has a reducing or depleting effect.

We must also consider the right-left predominance of the breath, which has its doshic action. Right nostril breathing energizes the pingala or solar nadi and increases pitta and fire. Left nostril breathing energizes the ida or lunar nadi and increases kapha and water. Balanced right and left nostril breathing helps vata.

Kapha is increased by breathing through the mouth, which has a cooling nature. However, mouth breathing mainly tends to increase waste kapha or mucus. For this reason it is generally not recommended, although a few special yogic pranayamas do employ it. Mouth breathing can keep the prana in the central channel or sushumna or in the sarasvati nadi, the channels of the mouth and throat, and work on udana vayu, aiding in the upward movement of prana.

Tonification and Reduction in Pranayama

Ayurvedic treatment strategies are either tonifying and building, called *brimhana*, or reducing and purifying, called *langhana*. Tonifying therapies increase body strength and weight and counter debilitating and wasting diseases. Reducing therapies reduce body weight and eliminate toxins, countering fevers and toxins.

Retention after deep inhalation increases the brimhana or tonifying effect of pranayama. It is useful for calming vata and building ojas. It has a stabilizing and grounding effect, giving strength to both body and mind.

Retention after exhalation increases the langhana or reducing aspect of pranayama. This is good for reducing kapha and increasing prana and has a detoxifying effect. It promotes the etheric or space-like nature of the mind, aiding in meditation, but it can aggravate vata if we hold the breath too long.

Types of Pranayama

To practice pranayama, sit in any comfortable sitting posture such as padmasana (lotus posture), siddhasana or sukhasana, or sit comfortably in a chair. Face either the north or the east. The room should be well ventilated but without direct exposure to the wind or temperature changes. The best time for practicing pranayama is the two-hour period before sunrise. Also good are sunrise and sunset and the time immediately before sleep (for a mild practice only).

Natural Breathing and So'ham Pranayama

The first place to start pranayama practice is with simple natural breathing. Allow your breath to deepen naturally and without effort. Mentally repeat the mantra *So* upon inhalation and *Ham* upon exhalation, meaning "That (the conscious spirit) am I." Become comfortable in this practice before attempting to manipulate the breath. So'ham pranayama should be performed with the ujjayi breath, breathing with a sound in the back of the throat.

Ujjayi Pranayama

Most forms of pranayama are done with the ujjayi breath. One breathes deeply, making a noticeable sound with the breath from the back of the throat. Ujjayi breathing has a heating effect. It reduces kapha and vata and improves agni, stimulating prana in the head, throat and heart. It should not be practiced during alternate nostril breathing, however, which should focus on the breath through the nostrils.

Alternate Nostril Breathing: Balancing Prana and Apana

Prana and apana relate to the right and left nostrils and their channels, the ida and pingala. They can be balanced by balancing the flow through these two nostrils.

This requires blocking the nostrils alternately during practice. First spread out the palm of your right hand. Turn down your index and middle fingers. Extend the other two fingers and the thumb. Place these on the bridge of the nose with the thumb on the right side and the extended fingers on the left. Use them to block the nostrils as needed. In its first form or solar breathing, inhale through the right or solar nostril and exhale through the left or lunar. Gradually increase the period of retention until sweating occurs. In lunar breathing, inhale through the left nostril and exhale through the right. This should be done to reduce body temperature and create coolness.

Alternate nostril breathing is the most important pranayama technique used in Ayurveda. The ida and pingala provide the main energy to the body and its organs on the right and left side. The right side of the trunk contains the main organs responsible for digestion, the liver, gall bladder, and right kidney, including a secondary solar chakra in the region of the liver. The right side of the body — along with the right eye, ear, nostril, hand, and foot — transmits a similar heating energy, providing acuity of perception and skill in action.

The organs responsible for nourishment, the heart and the stomach, as well as the left kidney, are located on the left side of the trunk, including a secondary lunar chakra in the region of the stomach. The left eye, ear, nostril, hand, and foot transmit a similar cooling energy providing emotional sensitivity, receptivity to nourishment, and rest.

Our breath predominates in one nostril at a time, alternating during different hours of the day. Right nostril breathing, which has a heating effect, occurs when the environment or bodily conditions are cool, or after eating when the body must produce heat to digest the food. When bodily and outside conditions are hot, breathing occurs mainly from the left nostril, which has a cooling effect as when we are resting or sleeping. Therefore patients suffering from diseases of cold like obesity, edema, muscle stiffness and paralysis should emphasize right nostril breathing.

On the other hand, patients suffering from diseases of heat, like fevers, wasting diseases, or paralysis along with loss of body weight, should emphasize left nostril breathing. Left nostril breathing is also useful in conditions of hyperactivity of the mind, including insomnia, restlessness, and nervous agitation. Right nostril breathing treats hypoactive conditions of the mind including sleepiness, dullness, and fatigue.

Another method used in ayurvedic treatment is to close off one nostril completely with a piece of cotton. To start off, do this practice only for a few minutes. Increase it slowly over a period of weeks until up to an hour or two. However, alternate nostril breathing is preferable to this if one can make the effort.

Alternate nostril breathing has the additional benefit that it is easier to control the breath and to make it longer or shorter. The nostril can be used like a straw to suck in air slowly, something regular nose or mouth breathing cannot do. For gaining control of the breath and purification of the channels there is no method better than alternate nostril breathing.

Alternate nostril breathing focuses the breath in the nostrils themselves, exercising their muscles and increasing the absorption of prana in the head. Ujjayi breath pranayama, on the other hand, draws the breath from the back of the sinuses, while mouth breathing draws air from the throat.

The Five Pranic Breaths

The following are a few simple exercises for developing the five pranas. They can be done by anyone. Doing them keeps all the pranas in balance.

1. Work with the Prana or Energizing Breath

The pranic breath is the breath in the head. It is energized through deep inhalation, drawing energy from above into the higher head and brain centers centered in the third eye.

Increasing the Pranic Breath: Take a series of sustained deep inhalations, drawing energy from the sky and space around you and bringing it through the head and senses into the third eye. Hold your energy in the third eye during retention as a ball of light and exhale through the third eye, spreading energy through all the senses. You can also do this practice with alternate nostril breathing, focusing on one side of the head at a time.

Visualize the prana coming in not only through the nostrils but also through the eyes, ears and mind, opening and purifying the channels and invigorating the entire brain and mind. Try to contact the prana at work in the head. Learn to see its scintillating series of electrical flashes, keeping the mind ever-thinking and senses ever-moving. More specifically, visualize prana like a revolving golden wheel with various spokes turning in the region of the head, setting off lightning currents that emerge through the sensory openings of the head and mouth. The prana breath is useful for treating all diseases of the mind, senses, head, brain and nervous system. It is particularly good for sinus allergies, head colds, and headaches. It aids in nervous exhaustion and brain fatigue. It provides a pranic bath to the brain, refreshing and revitalizing it for more productive mental activity.

2. Working with the Udana or Ascending Breath

The udana breath is the breath in the mouth. It is allied with thought, sound or mantra and the upward movement of the will.

Increasing the Udana Breath: Take a deep breath with the mouth and draw the energy into the throat chakra, holding it there upon retention. Upon exhalation loudly chant OM. Feel your energy rise and expand like a ball of light from the OM sound in the mouth to encompass the entire horizon and entire universe. Experience the throat as the center of cosmic sound, speech and vibration. Visualize udana like a deep blue lotus or a lotus-like pillar in the region of the throat and neck, holding your energy up and allowing it to ascend.

The udana breath treats all diseases of the throat region and vocal cords. It guards against sore throat, improves the voice, gives vitality and grants more strength. It helps anyone who needs greater powers of articulation and self-expression.

3. Working with the Vyana or Expanding Breath

The vyana breath is the breath in the heart that pervades the entire body and extends outward. Vyana breathing aims at opening the lung and heart region and from there expanding out to the rest of the body, the external world and the whole of life.

Increasing the Vyana Breath: Take a deep breath, preferably while standing, extending your arms as widely as possible and filling the heart and lungs with energy. Keep the arms wide apart during retention, visualizing your energy expanding from the heart through the blood stream to the entire body and limbs and out through the hands and feet into the external environment, extending all the way to the horizon. Close your arms upon exhalation, returning all energy to its source in the heart. Feel that your heart is the life-center of all creation. Visualize vyana like a revolving wheel, orange in color, spiraling outward as it turns into various rays.

The vyana breath treats all diseases of the circulatory and musculoskeletal systems. It is good for lung problems, heart disease, arthritis, asthma, and stress. It helps all those who need greater energy and coordination for physical exertion and movement.

4. Working with the Samana or Centering Breath

The samana breath is the breath in the navel or belly. Samana breathing aims at centering and balancing our energy.

Increase the Samana Breath: Visualize the energy from the entire universe and its many galaxies, stars and planets spiraling into your body from the distant horizon. Breathe deeply, bringing the breath down into the navel during inhalation, feeding the digestive fire. Hold the breath firmly in the navel during retention, letting the digestive fire blaze up. On exhalation, let the breath extend outward from the navel providing nourishment to all the tissues of your body and all the layers of the mind and heart. Visualize samana like a spiral of multi-colored energy turning inward into the navel and growing ever more small, concentrated and luminous, providing more stability and centeredness.

The samana breath treats all diseases of the digestive system, liver, gall bladder, stomach, and small intestine. It is particularly good for low appetite, poor absorption, and ulcers. It aids in homeostasis, balances metabolism, and has a balancing affect on both body and mind.

5. Working with the Apana or the Descending Breath

The apana breath is the breath in the root chakra that connects us with the earth and grounds us.

Increasing the Apana Breath: Take a deep breath, drawing your energy down to the base of the spine, feeling your body like a large and stable mountain. Hold the energy there on retention. Upon exhalation, ground the energy downward through your feet into the earth, allowing any physical or mental toxins to be released into the ground. View apana as a downward-facing dark blue triangle in the region of the lower abdomen, from which the energy moves downward in lightning flashes and grounds itself into the center of the earth below, where there dwells a special fire of strength and resistance.

The apana breath treats all diseases of the reproductive, urinary and excretory systems. It is good for constipation, diarrhea, menstrual problems and sexual debility. It strengthens the immune system, supports ojas, and aids in the prevention of disease.

6. Working with All Five Pranas

Do the exercises for the five pranas in order, about ten breaths for each prana. Then repeat the entire cycle from the apana breath up to the prana breath.

Forms of Nadi Pranayama

We can direct the breath through any of the fourteen nadis, not just the sushumna, ida or pingala. For purifying the senses we can direct the breath through any of the sensory nadis. We can practice the prana breath focusing on any of the nadis in the head. For such direction of prana to be efficacious, however, it should be done with a receptive mind open to the cosmic prana, not by mere personal effort.

One can direct the energy specifically by using the right nostril breath for right nadis and the left nostril breath for left nadis. For example, inhale through the right nostril, visualizing energy coming in through the right eye and its pusha nadi. Exhale through the left nostril, visualizing energy going out through the left eye and its gandhari nadi. This purifies the eyes and is good for all eye diseases.

Similarly, inhale through the right nostril, visualizing energy come in through the right ear and its payasvini nadi. Exhale through the left nostril, visualizing energy going out through the left ear and its shankhini nadi. This purifies the ears and is good for all ear diseases.

One can practice the vyana breath in the same way. Breathe deeply through the right nostril and fill the heart and lungs with the energy drawn in from the right hand and right leg and yashasvati nadi. Exhale through the left nostril and out through the left arm and leg to the palm of the left hand and sole of the left foot, the hastijihva nadi.

For the central nadis one can breathe through both nostrils. For the sarasvati nadi, the udana breath can be done by bringing the energy down from the tip of the tongue to the throat chakra on inhalation and from the throat chakra to the tip of the tongue on exhalation. One can similarly practice the vyana breath through the varuna or heart nadi. Draw the energy from the entire skin region back into the heart upon inhalation and out again upon exhalation.

One can practice the samana breath focusing on the vishvodhara nadi supplying all the organs of the digestive system. On inhalation, draw the energy from the digestive organs into the navel and back out again during exhalation. One can practice the apana breath focusing on either kuhu or alambusha to purify either the urinogenital or excretory organs. Again draw the energy down the channel during inhalation and out the channel during exhalation.

Sushumna Breathing

Sushumna breathing occurs when the prana stays in the sushumna or central channel. While this is very difficult to accomplish, we can simulate it in order to gradually set it in motion. Sushumna breathing proceeds mainly through udana, which allows our energy to move upward through the chakras. The udana breath also relates to the breath in the spine, which moves up and down. Spinal breathing helps promote sushumna breathing.

Increasing the Spinal Breath: Take a series of deep breaths visualizing the prana moving up the spine upon inhalation, having a cooling energy, and down the spine upon exhalation, having a heating energy. Use the mantra SO during inhalation and HAM during exhalation. Draw the breath up by degrees through the different pranic centers — from that of apana at the base of the spine to that of prana at the third eye. Increasing the spinal breath is the key to awakening the kundalini. Another method is to draw the prana up the spine through udana during inhalation and extend it out above the head during exhalation.

The Samadhi Breath

The samadhi breath is very subtle and arises when prana and apana are balanced. Ordinary respiration becomes suspended and an inner force of calm prana sustains both body and mind. In the samadhi breath, inhalation and exhalation become almost imperceptible. This occurs mainly through samana vayu functioning in the region of the heart and mind. The samana breath sustains metabolism and homeostasis on all levels, including on a cellular level. Samana allows for hibernation, suspending body functions while maintaining survival. It has a similar action in samadhi.

Method of Samadhi Breath: After a period of prolonged deep breathing, once the breath has become full, rest in the state of calmness of breath in which breathing is no longer necessary. Place your awareness in the heart, in the core or center of your being, and let all your energies return to it as their source. Let the breath flow imperceptibly like gentle waves on the sea. Experience the peace of mind that goes along with the peaceful breath. However, do not obstruct the natural flow of the breath. Should inhalation or exhalation be necessary, let them occur without strain or interference. The samadhi breath is the culmination of yoga practice and provides knowledge of the Self and the supreme peace of Brahman.

Heating Forms of Pranayama

Kapalabhati

This is also one of the procedures for cleansing the nasal passages in the head. The actual meaning is "what makes the head shine." First do a forceful exhalation a little deeper than ordinary breathing. At the same time, contract the front abdominal muscles suddenly and with a little force. Then inhale by simply relaxing the abdominal muscles. In this procedure do not do any retention of the breath. The beginner should start with eleven expulsions in each round. Each expiration stimulates the center of the abdomen and activates the prana. Kapalabhati also improves digestion and increases Agni.

Bhastrika

Sit in a comfortable posture. Close the left nostril as in right nostril breathing. Place your left hand on the left knee. Inhale and exhale through the right nostril without stopping, breathing deeply and forcefully at least ten times. Inhale and retain the breath as long as possible, then exhale through the left nostril, keeping the right nostril closed. In the second round, close the right nostril and breathe deeply and forcefully through the left nostril at least ten times.

Bhastrika is a very heating form of pranayama. It clears kapha from the head and chest and increases agni and prana. It counters cough and mucus and helps reduce body weight and fat. It aids in the awakening of kundalini. As it is a forceful practice it should be done with caution, particularly for weak constitutions, and care should be taken so that it does not aggravate pitta.

Cooling Forms of Pranayama

Shitali

Sit in a comfortable posture. Stick out your tongue and fold up its sides to form a long narrow tube like the beak of a crow. Narrow the passage further by pressing your lips around the tongue. Inhale slowly through the tongue, like sucking water. You will note a distinct cooling sensation. Fill the stomach with air and hold the breath as long as you can comfortably. Then exhale through the nostrils.

Shitali means "cooling" and more effectively counters diseases of heat than left nostril breathing. It counters thirst and builds the plasma. It is even used for high fevers and is an excellent practice for the summer. It is good for high blood pressure and hyperacidity. It is mainly for pitta types.

Sitkari

Follow the same procedure as shitali. However, while inhaling produce a sound like "see." Do not hold your breath but exhale immediately through the nostrils. Its benefits are similar to shitali. It clears heat from the head and cools the emotions.

Considerations for Pranayama Practice

A beginner should practice pranayama with an even ratio of inhalation, retention and exhalation, letting the breath naturally lengthen. Eventually one can extend the exhalation to twice as long as inhalation. After proficiency is gained, one should practice with a proportion of inhalation one, internal retention two, exhalation two, and external retention two. This requires some practice to achieve and should never be forced.

The ideal proportion is inhalation one, internal retention four, exhalation two, and external retention four, but only advanced practitioners can do this and it requires the development of much internal strength. In pranayama there should be no straining to achieve results but a natural development by letting go of strain and tension.

Pranayama and the Doshas

Vata: Practice mainly right nostril breathing in the morning for ten or fifteen minutes to stimulate energy. In the evening, do left nostril breathing to calm the mind and promote sleep. Bhastrika can be helpful when cold but should not be done excessively. Practice should be stopped if one feels dizzy or spaced out. Vatas should do the five prana breaths, focusing on the apana breath to keep grounded.

Pitta: Emphasize cooling pranayama. Do lunar or left nostril breathing, particularly in the evening or when feeling hot or irritable. Do shitali inhalation and sitkari exhalation if stronger cooling action is needed, particularly for heat in the head or overheated emotions. Pittas should do the breaths for the five pranas, particularly the vyana breath for expanding energy and releasing heat.

<u>Kapha</u>: Solar or right nostril breathing, which reduces excess kapha in the body, is best for kaphas, particularly in the morning, when kapha needs to be reduced. Bhastrika and kapalabhati are excellent, particularly when suffering from colds, congestion, lethargy or depression. Kapha types should do the five prana breaths, particularly the prana breath to clear kapha from the head and the vyana breath to clear it from the lungs.

Pranayama and the Paths of Yoga

All paths of yoga are based upon prana. Bhakti yoga or the yoga of devotion brings about pranic transformation by uniting us with the divine prana of love. Karma yoga or service is based upon alignment with the divine Will that gives us more prana, not only for outer actions but for inner development.

Classical yoga or Raja Yoga is based upon the control of mental activities (chitta-vrittis). The vibration of the mind (chitta-spanda) follows the vibration of prana (prana-spanda). Therefore, pranayama helps control the mind. Hatha yoga itself is mainly concerned with prana and asana occurs as an expression of prana. Even jnana yoga or the yoga of knowledge depends upon a strong will and concentration. Without a well-developed udana vayu, it cannot succeed. In the yoga of knowledge, the prana of inquiry must be created, which is to inquire into our true nature not merely mentally but in all of our daily activities. This requires that inquiry occurs through prana and not simply through the outer mind.

The *Vedas* say that we are all under the control of prana. Prana is the sun that imparts life and light to all and dwells within the heart as the Self of all creatures. We must open up to and welcome this greater force of prana, bringing it into our life and action. It is the energy through which all yoga proceeds.

16

Pratyahara

The Forgotten Limb of Yoga

Pratyahara itself is termed as Yoga,
as it is the most important limb in Yoga Sadhana.

SWAMI SHIVANANDA

Yoga is a vast system of spiritual practices for inner growth. To this end, the classical yoga system incorporates eight limbs, each with its own place and function. Of these, pratyahara is probably the least known. How many people, even yoga teachers, can define pratyahara? Have you ever taken a class in pratyahara? Have you ever seen a book on pratyahara? Can you think of several important pratyahara techniques? Do you perform pratyahara as part of your yogic practices? Yet unless we understand pratyahara, we are missing an integral aspect of yoga without which the system cannot work.

As the fifth of the eight limbs, pratyahara occupies a central place. Some yogis include it among the outer aspects of yoga, others with the inner aspects. Both classifications are correct, for pratyahara is the key between the outer and inner aspects of yoga; it shows us how to move from one to the other.

It is not possible to move directly from asana to meditation. This requires jumping from the body to the mind, forgetting what lies between. To make this transition, the breath and senses, which link the body and mind, must be brought under control

261

and developed properly. This is where pranayama and pratyahara come in. With pranayama we control our vital energies and impulses and with pratyahara we gain mastery over the unruly senses — both prerequisites to successful meditation.

What is Pratyahara?

The term *pratyahara* is composed of two Sanskrit words, *prati* and *ahara*. *Ahara* means "food," or "anything we take into ourselves from the outside." *Prati* is a preposition meaning "against" or "away." Pratyahara means literally "control of ahara," or "gaining mastery over external influences." It is compared to a turtle withdrawing its limbs into its shell — the turtle's shell is the mind and the senses are the limbs. The term is usually translated as "withdrawal from the senses," but much more is implied.

In yogic thought there are three levels of *ahara*, or food. The first is physical food that brings in the five elements necessary to nourish the body. The second is impressions, which bring in the subtle substances necessary to nourish the mind — the sensations of sound, touch, sight, taste, and smell. The third level of ahara is our associations, the people we hold at heart level who serve to nourish the soul and affect us with the gunas of sattva, rajas, and tamas.

Pratyahara is twofold. It involves withdrawal from wrong food, wrong impressions and wrong associations, while simultaneously opening up to right food, right impressions and right associations. We cannot control our mental impressions without right diet and right relationship, but pratyahara's primary importance lies in control of sensory impressions which frees the mind to move within.

By withdrawing our awareness from negative impressions, pratyahara strengthens the mind's powers of immunity. Just as a healthy body can resist toxins and pathogens, a healthy mind can ward off the negative sensory influences around it. If you are easily disturbed by the noise and turmoil of the environment around you, practice pratyahara. Without it, you will not be able to meditate.

There are four main forms of pratyahara: *indriya-pratyahara* — control of the senses; *prana- pratyahara* — control of prana; *karma-pratyahara* — control of action; and *mano-pratyahara* — withdrawal of mind from the senses. Each has its special methods.

1. Control of the Senses (Indriya-pratyahara)

Indriya-pratyahara, or control of the senses, is the most important form of pratyahara, although this is not something that we like to hear about in our mass media-oriented culture. Most of us suffer from sensory overload, the result of constant bombardment from television, radio, computers, newspapers, magazines, books — you name it. Our commercial society functions by stimulating our interest through the senses. We are constantly confronted with bright colors, loud noises and dramatic sensations. We have been raised on every sort of sensory indulgence; it is the main form of entertainment in our society.

The problem is that the senses, like untrained children, have their own will, which is largely instinctual in nature. They tell the mind what to do. If we don't discipline them, they dominate us with their endless demands. We are so accustomed to ongoing sensory activity that we don't know how to keep our minds quiet; we have become hostages of the world of the senses and its allurements. We run after what is appealing to the senses and forget the higher goals of life. For this reason, pratyahara is probably the most important limb of yoga for people today.

The old saying "the spirit is willing but the flesh is weak" applies to those of us who have not learned how to properly control our senses. Indriya-pratyahara gives us the tools to strengthen the spirit and reduce its dependency on the body. Such control is not suppression (which causes eventual revolt), but proper coordination and motivation.

Right Intake of Impressions

Pratyahara centers on the right intake of impressions. Most of us are careful about the food we eat and the company we keep, but we may not exercise the same discrimination about the impressions we take in from the senses. We accept impressions via the mass media that we would never allow in our personal lives. We let people into our houses through television and movies that we would never allow into our homes in real life! What kind of impressions do we take in every day? Can we expect that they will not have an effect on us? Strong sensations dull the mind, and a dull mind makes us act in ways that are insensitive, careless, or even violent.

According to Ayurveda, sensory impressions are the main food for the mind. The background of our mental field consists of our predominant sensory impressions. We see this when our mind reverts to the impressions of the last song we heard or the last movie we saw. Just as junk food makes the body toxic, junk impressions make the mind toxic. Junk food requires a lot of salt, sugar, or spices to make it palatable because it is largely dead food; similarly junk impressions require powerful dramatic impressions — sex and violence — to make us feel that they are real, because they are actually just colors projected on a screen.

We cannot ignore the role sensory impressions play in making us who we are, for they build up the subconscious and strengthen the tendencies latent within it. Trying to meditate without controlling our impressions pits our subconscious against us and prevents the development of inner peace and clarity.

Sensory Withdrawal

Fortunately we are not helpless before the barrage of sensory impressions. Pratyahara provides us many tools for managing them properly. Perhaps the simplest way to control our impressions is simply to cut them off, to spend some time apart from all sensory inputs. Just as the body benefits by fasting from food, so the mind benefits by fasting from impressions. This can be as simple as sitting to meditate with our eyes closed or taking a retreat somewhere free from the normal sensory bombardments, like at a mountain cabin. Also a "media fast," abstaining from television, radio, etc. can be a good practice to cleanse and rejuvenate the mind.

Yoni mudra is one of the most important pratyahara techniques for closing the senses. It involves using the fingers to block the sensory openings in the head — the eyes, ears, nostrils, and mouth — and allowing the attention and energy to move within. It is done for short periods of time when our prana is energized, such as immediately after practicing pranayama. (Naturally we should avoid closing the mouth and nose to the point at which we starve ourselves of oxygen.)

Another method of sense withdrawal is to keep our sense organs open but withdraw our attention from them. In this way we cease taking in impressions without actually closing off our sense organs. The most common method, *shambhavi mudra*, consists of sitting with the eyes open while directing the attention within, a technique used in several Buddhist systems of meditation as well. This redirection of the senses inward can be done with the other senses as well, particularly with the sense of hearing. It helps us control our mind even when the senses are functioning, as they are during the normal course of the day.

Focusing on Uniform Impressions

Another way to cleanse the mind and control the senses is to put our attention on a source of uniform impressions, such as gazing at the ocean or the blue sky. Just as the digestive system gets short-circuited by irregular eating habits and contrary food qualities, our ability to digest impressions can be deranged by jarring or excessive impressions. And just as improving our digestion may require going on a mono-diet, like the ayurvedic use of rice and mung beans (*kicharee*), so our mental digestion may require a diet of natural but homogeneous impressions. This technique is often helpful after a period of fasting from impressions.

Creating Positive Impressions

Another means of controlling the senses is to create positive, natural impressions. There are a number of ways to do this: meditating upon aspects of nature such as trees, flowers, or rocks, as well as visiting temples or other places of pilgrimage which are repositories of positive impressions and thoughts. Positive impressions can also be created by using incense, flowers, ghee lamps, altars, statues, and other artifacts of devotional worship.

Creating Inner Impressions

Another sensory withdrawal technique is to focus the mind on inner impressions, thus removing attention from external impressions. We can create our own inner impressions through the imagination or we can contact the subtle senses that come into play when the physical senses are quiet.

Visualization is the simplest means of creating inner impressions. In fact, most yogic meditation practices begin with some type of visualization, such as "seeing" a deity, a guru, or a beautiful setting in nature. More elaborate visualizations involve imagining deities and their worlds, or mentally performing rituals, such as offering imaginary flowers or gems to imagined deities. The artist absorbed in an inner landscape or the musician creating music are also performing inner visualizations. These are all forms of pratyahara because they clear the mental field of external impressions and create a positive inner impression to serve as the foundation of meditation. Preliminary visualizations are helpful for most forms of meditation and can be integrated into other spiritual practices as well.

Laya Yoga is the yoga of the inner sound and light current, in which we focus on subtle senses to withdraw us from the gross senses. This withdrawal into inner sound and light is a means of transforming the mind and is another form of indriya-pratyahara.

2. Control of the Prana (Prana-Pratyahara)

Control of the senses requires the development and control of prana because the senses follow prana (our vital energy). Unless our prana is strong we will not have the power to control the senses. If our prana is scattered or disturbed, our senses will also be scattered and disturbed.

Pranayama is a preparation for pratyahara. Prana is gathered in pranayama and withdrawn in pratyahara. Yogic texts describe methods of withdrawing prana from different parts of the body, starting with the toes and ending wherever we wish to fix our attention — the top of the head, the third eye, the heart or one of the other chakras.

Perhaps the best method of prana-pratyahara is to visualize

the death process, in which the prana, or the life-force, withdraws from the body, shutting off all the senses from the feet to the head. Ramana Maharshi achieved Self-realization by doing this when he was a mere boy of seventeen. Before inquiring into the Self, he visualized his body as dead, withdrawing his prana into the mind and the mind into the heart. Without such complete and intense pratyahara, his meditative process would not have been successful.

3. Control of Action (Karma-Pratyahara)

We cannot control the sense organs without also controlling the motor organs. In fact the motor organs involve us directly in the external world. The impulses coming in through the senses get expressed through the motor organs and this drives us to further sensory involvement. Because desire is endless, happiness consists not in getting what we want, but in no longer needing anything from the external world.

Just as the right intake of impressions gives control of the sense organs, right work and right action gives control of the motor organs. This involves karma yoga — performing selfless service and making our life a sacred ritual. Karma-pratyahara can be performed by surrendering any thought of personal rewards for what we do, doing everything as service to God or to humanity. The *Bhagavad Gita* says, "Your duty is to act, not to seek a reward for what you do." This is one kind of pratyahara. It also includes the practice of austerities that lead to control of the motor organs. For example, asana can be used to control the hands and feet, control which is needed when we sit quietly for extended periods of time.

4. Withdrawal of the Mind (Mano-Pratyahara)

The yogis tell us that mind is the sixth sense organ and

that it is responsible for coordinating all the other sense organs. We take in sensory impressions only where we place our mind's attention. In a way we are always practicing pratyahara. The mind's attention is limited and we give attention to one sensory impression by withdrawing the mind from other impressions. Wherever we place our attention, we naturally overlook other things.

We control our senses by withdrawing our mind's attention from them. According to the *Yoga Sutras II.54:* "When the senses do not conform with their own objects but imitate the nature of the mind, that is pratyahara." More specifically, it is mano-pratyahara — withdrawing the senses from their objects and directing them inward to the nature of the mind, which is formless. Vyasa's commentary on the *Yoga Sutra* notes that the mind is like the queen bee and the senses are the worker bees. Wherever the queen bee goes, all the other bees must follow. Thus mano-pratyahara is less about controlling the senses than about controlling the mind, for when the mind is controlled, the senses are automatically controlled.

We can practice mano-pratyahara by consciously withdrawing our attention from unwholesome impressions whenever they arise. This is the highest form of pratyahara and the most difficult; if we have not gained proficiency in controlling the senses, motor organs, and pranas, it is unlikely to work. Like wild animals, prana and the senses can easily overcome a weak mind, so it is usually better to start first with more practical methods of pratyahara.

Pratyahara and the Other Limbs of Yoga

Pratyahara is related to all the limbs of yoga. All of the other limbs — from asana to samadhi — contain aspects of pratyahara. For example, in the sitting poses, which are the most important aspect of asana, both the sensory and motor organs are controlled. Pranayama contains an element of pratyahara as we draw our attention inward through the breath. Yama and niyama contain various principles and practices, like non-violence and contentment, that help us control the senses. In other words, pratyahara provides the foundation for the higher practices of yoga and is the basis for meditation. It follows pranayama (or control of prana) and, by linking prana with the mind, takes it out of the sphere of the body.

Pratyahara is also linked with dharana. In pratyahara we withdraw our attention from ordinary distractions. In dharana we consciously focus that attention on a particular object, such as a mantra. Pratyahara is the negative and dharana the positive aspect of the same basic function.

Many of us find that even after years of meditation practice we have not achieved all that we expected. Trying to practice meditation without some degree of pratyahara is like trying to gather water in a leaky vessel. No matter how much water we bring in, it flows out at the same rate. The senses are like holes in the vessel of the mind. Unless they are sealed, the mind cannot hold the nectar of truth. Anyone whose periods of meditation alternate with periods of sensory indulgence is in need of pratyahara.

Pratyahara offers many methods of preparing the mind for meditation. It also helps us avoid environmental disturbances that are the source of psychological pain. Pratyahara is a marvelous tool for taking control of our lives and opening up to our inner being. It is no wonder some great yogis have called it "the most important limb of yoga." We should all remember to include it in our practice.

Pratyahara and Ayurveda

Pratyahara, as right management of the mind and senses, is essential and good for all constitutional types. It is the most important factor for mental nutrition. However, it is most essential for those with a vata constitution who tend towards imbalanced or excessive sensory and mental activity. All vata types should practice some form of pratyahara daily. Their restless vata distracts the senses, disturbs the motor organs and prana, and makes the mind restless. Pratyahara reverse harmful vata and turns it into a positive force of prana.

Kapha types, on the other hand, generally suffer from too little activity, including on a sensory level. They may slip into tamasic patterns of being lazy, watching television or sitting around the house. They need more mental stimulation and benefit from sensory activity of a higher nature, like visualizations of various types.

Pitta types generally have more control of the senses than the others and incline toward martial-type activities in which they discipline the body and the senses. They need to practice pratyahara as a means of relaxing the personal will and letting the divine will work through them.

Pratyahara and Disease

Ayurveda recognizes that the inappropriate use of the senses is one of the main causes of disease.[38] All mental disease is connected with the intake of unwholesome impressions. Pratyahara therefore is an important first step in treating all mental disorders. Similarly it is very helpful in treating nervous system disorders, particularly those that arise through hyperactivity. Most of the time we overly express our emotions, which loses tremendous energy. Pratyahara teaches us to hold our energy within and not disperse it unnecessarily. This conserved energy can be drawn upon for creative, spiritual or healing purposes as needed and can provide the extra power to do the things that are really important to us.

Physical disease mainly arises from taking in unwholesome food. Pratyahara affords us control of the senses so that we do not crave wrong food. When the senses are controlled, everything is controlled and no wrong or artificial cravings can arise. That is why Ayurveda emphasizes right use of the senses as one of the most important factors in right living and disease prevention.

17

Mantra Purusha

The Person of Sound

Repetition of mantra is the best means
for the alleviation of all diseases.

KARMATHAGURU

I f we carefully examine all the different yogic paths from
devotion and knowledge to hatha and raja yogas, we will
discover that mantra is the most common yogic practice.
We could say that yoga is mantra. While the asanas or postures
for the body may be more evident, mantras are equally important as postures for the mind. Just as asana gives health and
flexibility to the body, so mantra provides well-being and adaptability to the mind.

Mantra, energized sound or the sacred word, is the basis of
all religious traditions, scriptures and prayers. In one form or
another, it is the key religious practice of humanity. As we are
constantly either talking to others or speaking to ourselves
through our thoughts, we should learn to employ the power of
sound and the Word to master this main activity of our lives.
This is the basis of mantra yoga.

Mantra is also the main practice that links yoga and Ayurveda.
The two basic treatment methods of Ayurveda are herbs for the
body and mantras for the mind. Whereas yoga employs mantra
for self-development, Ayurveda uses it for self-healing. Mantra

is the main tool for working on the mind. Its influence extends to the deepest level of our consciousness. Mantra, repeated mentally, cleanses the causal body or samskaric field of the soul and helps alter subconscious habits and afflictions.

On the other hand, mantra, as spoken or chanted, is an important tool for healing the subtle body and clearing our field of impressions. Mantra can be used to direct the healing power of prana, which it carries. Prana has its own sound or mantric power that we can learn to master and direct at will through the right use of speech and sound. I have dealt with prana mantra at some length in my other books, particularly *Ayurveda and the Mind*. Here I will add an important teaching on mantra through which we can link together physical and psychological practices. The chapter also contains a key to the pronunciation of Sanskrit.

Mantra Purusha

Sound is the original form of all energy. Space, which ultimately is consciousness, gives rise to energy which is prana or life. Sound is the mental aspect of prana. All aspects of the mind, from the outer to the inner, have their corresponding sound vibration. The mind is composed of thoughts, which are words and sounds. Each person's mind has its own sound pattern or mantra. The soul itself has its own mantric vibration; when we learn it, we can awaken all the powers within.

Sound always has a referent, an object for which it is the name. Each sound is a name which reflects the idea behind the sound. All names link us to the being or object that they designate. Sound is a means of directing awareness through the name to a particular object. Along with awareness always goes energy or prana. Hence, through mantra we can direct the energy of consciousness and prana and link it up with whatever we seek.

This is the importance of prayer or speaking to the divine, through which we can receive divine grace. We can even speak to the limbs and organs of the body. Mantra can direct a healing energy to them and awaken the organic intelligence that is present in the cells.

The human being is a creation of sound which creates our different bodies, starting with the causal body. The causal body, soul or deeper mind is our aspect of the divine Word. The Creator breathes this divine Word into the soul as its immortal life. This Word is the vibration of cosmic consciousness which is the origin of time, space, intelligence and prana. It forms the ideal pattern or dharma behind our soul's existence.

The subtle body is also a creation of sound. Sound is the sense quality of the element of ether that generates and sustains the field of impressions that is the subtle body. Prana itself is unmanifest sound, which we hear through the natural sound of the breath. Even the physical body is shaped by sound. Speech, the breath, and the pumping of the heart create the rhythm through which the physical body functions.

The human body, therefore, is a sound body and we can work on its energies through sound alone. The human body can be represented by the letters of the Sanskrit alphabet, called the *Mantra Purusha* or "person of sound." In this regard, the sixteen Sanskrit vowels make up the head of the Mantra Purusha; the five sets of five consonants, twenty five in all, make up the four limbs and the trunk. The five semi-vowels and four "s" and "h" sounds make up the tissues, prana and mind.

Vowels have an open sound and do not depend upon a consonant for their pronunciation. Therefore they represent mind and spirit, the formless aspect of reality that works through the head and the senses. Consonants are dependent sounds, requiring a vowel for their pronunciation. Therefore they represent matter and form, which is expressed in the body through the trunk and limbs that give us a shape and allow us to function in the material world.

Semi-vowels, as the name indicates, are intermediate sounds between vowels and consonants, half-vowels or half-consonants. "S" and "h" sounds are also intermediate in nature as they can be held longer than ordinary consonants. Semi-vowels govern the outer tissues and the elements of the body. "S" and "h" sounds govern the deeper tissues, breath (prana) and mind and possess a special power to create heat. These are the intermediate factors through which the spirit (head), represented by the vowels, creates and governs matter (body) represented by the consonants. In other words, these correlations are not merely incidental but reflect the universal energetics of sound. I have also listed their planetary equivalents. Note Appendix 3 for Sanskrit Pronunciation Table.

16 Sounds in the head and senses, Sun

अं	aṃ	Top of Head	आं	āṃ	Forehead
इं	iṃ	Right Eye	ईं	īṃ	Left Eye
उं	uṃ	Right Ear	ऊं	ūṃ	Left Ear
ऋं	r̥ṃ	Right Cheek	ॠं	r̥̄ṃ	Left Cheek
ऌं	l̥ṃ	Right Nostril	ॡं	l̥̄ṃ	Left Nostril
एं	eṃ	Upper Lips	ऐं	aiṃ	Lower Lips
ओं	oṃ	Upper Teeth	औं	auṃ	Lower Teeth
अं	aṃ	Top of palate	अः	aḥ	Bottom of palate

25 Sounds in the Trunk and Limbs

Right Side, Mars		Left Side, Venus		
क'	kaṃ	च'	caṃ	Shoulder Joint
ख'	khaṃ	छ'	chaṃ	Elbow Joint
ग'	gaṃ	ज'	jaṃ	Wrist Joint
''	ghaṃ	झ'	jhaṃ	Base of Fingers
ङ'	ṅaṃ	ञ'	ñaṃ	Tip of Fingers
Right Side, Mercury		Left Side, Jupiter		
ट'	ṭaṃ	त'	taṃ	Hip Joint
ठ'	ṭhaṃ	थ'	thaṃ	Knee Joint
ड'	ḍaṃ	द'	daṃ	Ankle
ढ'	ḍhaṃ	ध'	dhaṃ	Base of Toes
ण'	ṇaṃ	न'	naṃ	Tip of Toes
Trunk, Saturn				
प'	paṃ	Right Abdomen		
फ'	phaṃ	Lower Abdomen		
ब'	baṃ	Left Abdomen		
भ'	bhaṃ	Base of Throat		
म'	maṃ	Heart		

Nine Sounds of Tissues, Moon

य'	yaṃ	Plasma	Heart or Air Chakra
र'	raṃ	Blood	Navel or Fire Chakra
ळ'	laṃ	Muscle	Root or Earth Chakra
व'	vaṃ	Fat	Sex or Water Chakra
श'	śaṃ	Bone	Retention of Breath
ष'	ṣaṃ	Marrow	Retention of Breath
स'	saṃ	Reproductive	Inhalation
ह'	haṃ	Prana	Throat or Ether Chakra/ Exhalation
क्ष'	kṣaṃ	Mind	Third Eye

These mantras relate to prime *marmas* or sensitive points on the body, the sensory openings and the joints where prana is held. By repeating the sounds of the Sanskrit alphabet according to their specific place in the body, we can energize the entire body with consciousness and prana and relieve any obstructions in these regions.

The Mantra Purusha consonants are particularly useful in treating arthritis or other musculoskeletal disorders, using the mantras for the limbs and trunk. We can visualize the prana radiating out from each of these positions along with the inner repetition of the mantra. In this way the Mantra Purusha becomes a form of pranayama or expansion of the life-force.

These Mantra Purusha vowels treat sensory disorders and other diseases of the head, mind and brain. The mantra **aṃ** works on the higher aspects of the mind. The mantra **āṃ** works on the perceptual side of the mind. The mantras **iṃ** and **īṃ** improve vision, relative to the right and left eye. The mantras **uṃ** and **ūṃ** strengthen the right and left ears. The mantra **OM** in particular strengthens the mouth and the voice.

The mantras for the tissues and chakras are of particular importance and can be used for energizing the body from within and through the spine and the chakras. The Mantra Purusha is also useful for pratyahara. We can use these sounds to withdraw the prana from the different parts of the body and place it in the mind alone. Using the Mantra Purusha, we can gain power over our limbs, senses, prana and mind, learning to switch energy and attention off and on to the different parts of the body.

Mantra Purusha Energization and Relaxation Exercises

One should recite the Mantra Purusha daily before meditation, first using it to energize all the parts of the body and then using it to calm them and place the body in a state of peace and receptivity. This is a complete energization exercise for the mind, like doing the sun salutation for the body.

Recite the Mantra Purusha sounds, starting with the head, to energize all these parts of the body with prana. This is a mantra pranayama exercise.

Recite the Mantra Purusha sounds, withdrawing prana from all these parts of the body, and leave the energy in the third eye. This is a mantra pratyahara exercise.

The Mantra Purusha is a complete set of postures for the mind and prana.

Other Ways to Use the Sanskrit Alphabet

The Sanskrit alphabet is the garland of letters that the Goddess, the Yoga Shakti or Kundalini, wears. One way to awaken this energy is to recite these letters in order from the vowels to the consonants and semi-vowels.

Another way is to recite them relative to the chakras. Each letter corresponds to a petal of the chakras. In this method one starts with the throat chakra, which corresponds with the vowels, and moves down from there.

One recites the alphabet from the throat chakra down to the base of the spine and then up to the third eye. This draws the sound and prana current down to the base of the spine to awaken kundalini. The throat marks *vaikhari* or the audible stage of speech. The heart marks *madhyama* or the pranic stage of speech. The navel marks *pashyanti* or the mental (illumined) form of speech. The root chakra marks *para* or the supreme level of speech, which is beyond words. In this regard the higher power of speech lays hidden below in the root chakra as kundalini shakti. Note the following table for the order of the letters.

Sanskrit Alphabet through the Chakras

1. Throat Chakra: 16 Vowels

aṃ, āṃ, iṃ, īṃ, uṃ, ūṃ, ṛṃ, ṝṃ, ḷṃ, ḹṃ, eṃ, aiṃ, oṃ, auṃ, aṃ, aḥ

2. Heart Chakra: first 12 Consonants

kaṃ, khaṃ, gaṃ, ghaṃ, ṅaṃ, caṃ, chaṃ, jaṃ, jhaṃ, ñaṃ, ṭaṃ, ṭhaṃ

3. Navel Chakra: next 10 Consonants

ḍaṃ, ḍhaṃ, ṇaṃ, taṃ, thaṃ, daṃ, dhaṃ, naṃ, paṃ, phaṃ

4. Sex Chakra: next 3 Consonants and first 3 semi-vowels

baṃ, bhaṃ, maṃ, yaṃ, raṃ, laṃ

5. Root Chakra: next 4 semi vowels

vaṃ, śaṃ, ṣaṃ, saṃ

6. Third Eye: Final 2 semi-vowels

haṃ, kṣaṃ

Important Bija Mantras

OM

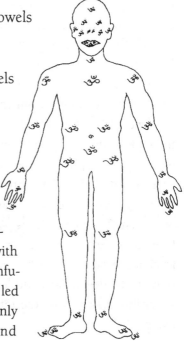

Om is the most important of all mantras. All mantras generally begin and often also end with Om. However, there is much confusion about Om. Some people are led to believe that Om is a mantra only for monks and renunciates and should not be repeated by those who still work in the world. This is not entirely correct. Chanting **Om** by itself is generally a practice more for those who want to renounce everything and directly transcend, but **Om** can be safely combined with other mantras and will enhance their power, even those mantras aimed at helping us in our outer lives.

The Four Great Goddess Mantras

There are four great Goddess mantras that govern the prime forms of energy as magnetic force, electrical force, heat, and delight.

HRĪM

Hrīm is the prime mantra of the Great Goddess and ruler of the worlds and holds all her creative and healing powers. **Hrīm** governs over the cosmic magnetic energy and the power of the soul and causal body. It awakens us at a soul or heart level, connecting us to Divine forces of love and attraction. **Hrīm** is the mantra of the Divine Maya that destroys the worldly maya. It has a solar quality to it but more of a dawn-like effect. It is charming and alluring, yet purifying . Through it we can control the illusion power of our own minds.

KRĪM

Krīm is the great mantra of Kali, the Goddess of energy and transformation. It governs over prana as lightning or electrical energy. Through **Krīm** ojas is transformed into not only tejas but prana. **Krīm** grants all spiritual faculties and powers — from the arousing of kundalini to opening the third eye. It has a special power relative to the lower chakras, which it can both stimulate and transform. It helps awaken and purify the subtle body. As a mantra of work and transformation **Krīm** is the mantra of Kriya Yoga, the Yoga of practice. It is the main mantra of the Yoga Shakti. As it is a strong mantra it should be used with care.

HUṂ

Huṃ is a mantra of the inner fire or thermogenic force. It both calls the divine down into us and offers our soul upward to the Divine for transformation in the sacred fire of awareness. It is a Shiva mantra but also a mantra of Chandi, the fierce form of Kali. It is used to destroy negativity and creates great passion and vitality. As a powerful mantra it should also be used carefully. Yet it can be used in a more gentle manner to invoke divine grace and protection. Through it we can offer ourselves or our afflictions into the Divine for purification and transformation.

ŚRĪM

Śrīm is a mantra of love, devotion and beauty, relating to Lakshmi, the Goddess of Beauty and divine grace. Yet Śrīm works at a deeper level than merely to give us the good things of life, including health. It takes us to the heart and gives faith and steadiness to our emotional nature. Śrīm allows us to surrender to, take refuge in, or be immersed in whatever we offer the mantra to. It is the mantra of beauty and delight and has a pleasing lunar quality. It also relates to the head and can be used to flood the senses with divine beauty and delight. It promotes health and aids in fertility and rejuvenation. It is one of the softest and safest mantras to use.

These four mantras can be used together with **OM: OM HRĪM KRĪM HUṂ ŚRĪM**! This brings about an integral development of body, mind and soul.

18

Meditation and the Mind

Yoga and knowledge are the two methods for
dissolving the disturbances of the mind.
Yoga is control of the movements of the mind.
Knowledge (Jnana) is clear observation of them.

LAGHU YOGA VASISHTA V.9.72

Meditation is the essential and culminating practice of the greater system of yoga. Of the eight limbs of yoga, the three inner aspects — *dharana* (concentration), *dhyana* (meditation) and *samadhi* (absorption) — refer specifically to the practice of meditation. Ayurveda as mind-body medicine promotes meditation as one of its main therapies. Much of Ayurveda's popularity comes from its emphasis on meditation and related techniques of mantra and pranayama.

Yet meditation proper is a very subtle state that is hard to reach. It requires that we first harmonize the body, prana and senses. Meditation is not just a matter of closing one's eyes and sitting silently. An understanding of meditation rests upon understanding the mind. To approach the subject of meditation let us first look at the mind and how it works.

Mind and Body

Both mind and body are composed of the five elements. The mind, however, is made up of a mental rather than a physical form of the elements. Mind and body have opposite elemental structures. The body is composed of the heavy elements of earth and water (kapha) which make up the form of the body and its various tissues. Body functions proceed through the lighter elements and doshas of pitta (fire) and vata (air), with fire determining all digestive processes and air determining the transmission of nerve and brain impulses.

On the other hand, the mind is made up of the lighter elements of air and ether (vata), as it is both pervasive and mobile. Its functions proceed through the heavier elements of fire, water and earth (pitta and kapha). Fire affords perception to the mind, water gives it emotion, and earth connects the mind with the body.

The mind in general is like the wind or vata dosha, which is similarly marked by pervasiveness and movement. Like vata, the mind is composed of the air and ether elements but at a more subtle level. The mind is like ether in substance, formless and all-pervading. Wherever we place our attention, there our mind already is. The mind is like air in motion, quick, penetrating and ever shifting and changing, lightning fast and unpredictable.

COMPARATIVE ELEMENTS OF BODY AND MIND

Body		Mind	
Substance	Earth and Water	Substance	Air and Ether
Kapha	Blood and Flesh	Vata	Sensitivity and Movement
	Functions		Functions
Pitta	Fire - Digestion	Pitta	Fire - Reason and Perception
Vata	Air and Ether	Kapha	Water and Earth
	Prana and Brain		Emotion and Identification with Body

Mind and Prana

Mind and prana always go together. Wherever we place our attention, there our energy naturally follows. Our attention itself directs a current of energy. Similarly, whatever motivates our energy and vitality, like hunger or thirst, engages our attention. Mind and prana are two sides of the same phenomenon, the two wings of the bird of the soul.

Though prana is generally grosser than the mind, there is a prana in the mind itself, the mind's own energy and vitality. Similarly there is a mind or consciousness in the workings of prana, the intelligence of the life-force. There is always some aspect of mind in prana and some aspect of prana in mind. Prana is inherently a power of intelligence or mind; mind is inherently a power of action and expression of prana.

Prana, like the mind, is also vata in nature and composed of the air and ether elements. But there is a difference. Prana has more of the air element and the mind has more of space or the ether element. Prana is more active, like air, while the mind is more receptive and observant, like space. In this regard we could say that the ether aspect of prana is the mind, while the air aspect of mind is prana.[39]

Doshic Types and the Levels of the Mind

The mind as a whole, what is called *chitta* or *antahkarana* in yogic literature, is in the sphere of vata, similarly composed of air and ether elements. However, the mind is subtler than vata, just as it is subtler than prana from which vata springs.

Vata imparts speed and energy to the mind. Vata types have quicker minds than other types and greater facility on all levels of mental activity — from sensory perception to deep formless perception. They are good at making connections (air) and have broad comprehension (space). Their minds are very active, always striving to go everywhere and comprehend everything. Because of vata's connection with the mind in general, vata types are more likely to suffer from mental and psychological disturbances. Their minds are immediately and strongly affected by whatever they do. In the same way, most mental and nervous system disorders are likely to cause vata aggravation. However, the mind has its pitta and kapha sides as well. As a power of light and illumination, the mind relates to pitta. For this reason the mind is sometimes identified with fire. Pitta more specifically is the perceptive power of the mind, while background mental field is more vata in nature. We could say that the mind is vata (airy) in nature but pitta (fiery) in its application. The mind has its special power of sight, the mind's eye or third eye that relates to fire. The pitta or fiery side of the mind is discrimination, reason and insight (buddhi), which is also the power of mental digestion. Pitta types are highly intelligent and discerning. They usually have the best mental focus of all the types, with sharp and clear thinking.

The kapha side of the mind is its feeling capacity from which arises emotion, love and attachment. These are connected to the senses and the outer or form aspect of the mind (manas). The kapha side of the mind is the most outward and material, just as kapha is the most material of the doshas. Yet there is a higher kapha side to the mind. The inner mind or heart has its feeling side as well, like love, the most important Kapha feeling. The bliss itself at the core of the mind is the highest form of kapha.

Meditation According to Ayurveda

Meditation is our ability to contact our true Self and consciousness (Atman or Purusha) which is the source of life and intelligence. Conversely, meditation is the ability to clear out the negative aspects of our consciousness, harmful subconscious habits and impulses that cause pain and suffering. Meditation helps promote our highest impulses and also roots out those which are harmful and intractable.

Meditation involves placing the mind in a calm and concentrated state in which our mental energies can be renewed and transformed. Such a definition deals with meditation in the broadest sense, which includes the many helpful techniques of mantra, pranayama and visualization. Yet whatever meditation techniques we employ should be used as aids to return our consciousness to its original peaceful and silent state, at which stage we can set the techniques aside and rest in the harmony of our true Nature. This is called "abiding in the Self." It is the natural state of meditation, which is the real goal of all meditative striving.

Meditation is an important tool in Ayurveda for healing the mind, but its benefits extend to the body as well. It reduces the psychological root or complications of the disease process, which always exist to some degree. Ayurveda recommends meditation for treating specific diseases, particularly psychological disorders in which meditation may be the primary therapy. Ayurveda also prescribes meditation as part of its lifestyle regimens both for health maintenance and life-enhancement. There are many types of meditation in ayurvedic and yogic thought. Here we will propose an ayurvedic rationale and application for meditation relative to the doshas, the gunas and functions of the mind.

Because of the mind's connection with prana, the role of pranic practices in meditation cannot be ignored. Because of prana's connection to food, the physical body cannot be forgotten either. The ayurvedic approach to meditation is always integral and includes body, breath and senses.

Meditation as a Therapy (*Dhyana Chikitsa*)

Meditation is an important therapy for psychological and nervous disorders, from simple insomnia to severe emotional disturbances. It is useful in chronic and debilitating diseases like allergies or arthritis, in which stress or hypersensitivity of the nervous system are involved. Western research has found meditation to be very helpful in treating heart disease. The heart is the seat of consciousness in Vedic thought. This is not simply the physical heart but our inner core of feeling and knowing beyond the sensory mind. Disturbances in our consciousness are reflected in problems with the heart, including on a physical level. Calming the mind and strengthening the heart go together.

Meditation helps us deal with pain and should be taught to all patients suffering from painful diseases, whether chronic or acute. We can take our mind off the pain of disease and place our attention in a mantra or in the witnessing mind. Meditation is most important in severe or terminal diseases where death may be near. It prepares the person for the transition into the next life. In fact, meditation helps all of us detach from the body. Attachment to the body is the main cause of physical, psychological and spiritual pain. Removing this attachment is the ultimate cure for all diseases or the way to transcend them if we cannot avoid them.

Some spiritual teachers hold that changing one's thoughts can cure all diseases, even terminal illnesses. Ayurveda has two qualifications on this. The first is the movement of time. Certain diseases born of time and aging can be postponed but not eliminated altogether. That is why we all must eventually die. The second is karma. We function according to certain karmas that keep us in this world for a particular period of time. Once our karma is completed, we must move on and sometimes disease is the means to do this. We must never forget that physical life is only one level of existence for the soul, a temporary journey. Therefore, we need not cling to physical existence but should strive to fulfill our purpose here and then continue on.

However, all forms of meditation are not good for everyone, any more than all foods or herbs are. For this reason Ayurveda recommends the proper lifestyle and an integral approach to meditation that considers both our different faculties and the nature of the individual.

Background of Meditation

Meditation should be grounded in a proper lifestyle, particularly a sattvic diet, sattvic impressions and sattvic associations. Without these we may not be capable of real meditation, even if we want to practice it. In such cases the background for meditation should be taught along with the practice of meditation. Ayurvedic life-regimens provide this.

Generally one begins a meditation session with a formal practice, employing techniques like prayer, mantra, pranayama or visualization. Then formless meditation can proceed, like sitting in silence, practicing self-inquiry or performing devotional meditation (meditating on God). If we merely sit silently without using any tools to calm the mind first, we may simply get lost in our own thoughts and end up more confused and disturbed.

Meditation, particularly of a passive nature, opens up the subconscious mind. If we are not ready to handle it, this can cause complications. People who are emotionally disturbed, particularly when vata is aggravated, are most vulnerable. For this reason mantra may be better than silent meditation, at least in the beginning. Silent meditation is expansive, but for the mind to truly expand it must first be concentrated. This is why concentration exercises usually precede meditation.

Ayurveda tries to affirm the natural meditational inclinations of people. There are many paths, teachings and traditions of meditation that have their value and relevance to different individuals and cultures. However, sometimes the meditation practices people follow may not be helping them from an ayurvedic standpoint. Vata people may not benefit from trying to space their minds out further. Pitta people may get disturbed by too focused or critical a meditative approach. Kapha types may have kapha increased by too emotional forms of meditation. In such instances Ayurveda may recommend that the nature of one's meditation changes.

Meditation and Prayer

People in the West are more familiar with prayer than meditation. Prayer is a general term and many types of it exist, but the term usually refers to an active form of meditation in which we project an intention — calling on God to help us or our loved ones in some way. Ayurveda uses prayer (*prarthana*) along with mantra and meditation. Generally mantra is energized prayer, a prayer or wish yogically directed by special sound patterns or vibrations of the cosmic Word. Meditation is a silent or contemplative form of prayer in which there may not be any movement of thought or intention.

Ayurvedic doctors use prayer or the direction of positive energies and intentions to treat diseases. This includes channeling the healing force of the divine or the powers of great teachers, avatars and gurus. Prayer as the giving of good wishes is necessary to create the proper psychic environment for healing to take place. It can be used along with the subtle healing modalities of Ayurveda of aromas, gems, mantras, and rituals.

Affirmation and Visualization

The use of affirmations goes along with prayer. Affirmations can be employed to emphasize our relationship with the divine or our own inner healing powers. Many people suffer from negative thoughts about themselves, particularly vata types who are often trapped in self-doubt. Affirmations can be very strengthening in such conditions.

Yet affirmations should lead to action and not substitute for it. For example, to do anything in life, like climbing a mountain, requires a belief that one can do it and a positive intention to make the effort. But one still has to climb the mountain and cannot use the affirmation as an excuse for inaction. Affirmations should be ways of attuning our will to the divine will and to our higher purpose in life that we follow with our behavior. Visualization goes along with prayer and meditation. We can visualize the healed or improved condition that we wish to achieve, like visualizing the lungs clear and open and full of energy for one suffering from chronic congestion. We can direct prana or healing energy to those who are sick or to the parts of our own body that need improvement. Such visualizations may employ certain colors and mantras or be directed along with the breath. Visualizations can also be of deities or beautiful scenes in nature to clear the mental field.

Samkalpa: The Power of the Will in Healing and Transformation

Samkalpa means will and motivation. It is the most important activity of the mind on all levels which is always engaged in the projection of intentions. We are the result of our samkalpas, much like the old proverb: "As a man wishes in his heart, so is he." We create ourselves and our karma through our samkalpas or intentions at a heart level. Samkalpa is the main mental action for creating samskaras, the deep-seated conditionings behind the mind and heart.

Yoga cultivates the will or samkalpa for Self-realization. Ayurveda cultivates the will or samkalpa of healing. Whatever action we do should be preceded by a samkalpa or statement of intentions: "I intend to do the following action (in the following manner for a specific period of time) in order to produce the following result."

Samkalpa is like a plan or a strategy. We do something in a certain way to arrive at a certain goal. The result that we gain tells us the nature and the value of our action. No action is done without the seeking of some sort of result. This result depends upon the intention behind the action, not simply the externalities of what we do. Higher or spiritual actions seek a result that is not ego-bound, like the development of consciousness and the alleviation of suffering for all beings. Lower actions reflect ego desires — to get what we want; to accomplish, achieve or gain for ourselves in some way or another. Spiritual samkalpas direct us within and help liberate the soul. Ego-based samkalpas direct us without and bind us further to the external world.

Samkalpa implies not only developing our own will but also allying our will with the forces that can help it achieve its aim. Therefore it involves a seeking of help, blessings or guidance. Samkalpas are generally projected as various affirmations and vows.

Yogic Samkalpas

Yogic samkalpas are spiritually based. They consist of the intention that one will perform various yogic practices in order to grow spiritually and advance the spiritual cause in the world. Below are a few typical such Samkalpas.

- Bhakti Yoga or Devotional Samkalpas:
  "OM! I will perform the following yogic practices as an offering to the Divine Beloved. May all the divine powers bless me in this endeavor!"

- Jnana Yoga or Wisdom-based Samkalpas:
  "OM! I will perform the following meditations to gain knowledge of God and the higher Self. May God and the great teachers aid me in this effort!"

- Karma Yoga or Service Samkalpas:
  "OM! I will perform the following actions as a service to God and to living beings in order to help alleviate suffering!"

Ayurvedic Samkalpas

Ayurveda uses samkalpa as a tool for healing. All healing practices should begin with the proper intention in both the patient and the therapist. The appropriate samkalpa sets the stage for healing processes to function and creates clarity in both the patient and the therapist as to the results that are being sought.

- Samkalpa for Patients:
  "OM! I seek to heal myself through natural and spiritual methods in order to create optimal health and vitality to develop my spiritual life and fulfill my dharma for the good of all!"
- Samkalpa for Therapists:
  "OM! I seek to aid in the healing of this patient through natural and spiritual methods in order to alleviate their suffering and help awaken human beings to their true purpose in life. May all the forces of healing in the universe support me in this endeavor!"

Aspects of Meditation

Meditation is a way of life that rests on certain procedures. One does not simply sit down to meditate suddenly all at once, any more than one simply, without training, takes up a brush and begins to paint as an accomplished artist.

General Format of Meditation

1. Sit in a comfortable posture with an erect spine, which can be a specific yoga posture like the lotus pose, or sit in a chair for those who cannot do this. Without a comfortable and re-laxed posture, it is very difficult to meditate.

2. Energize the breath through pranayama. This directs our energy internally, which gives us more power for meditation. It

can be done by any form of appropriate pranayama.

3. Hold a visualization for a few minutes to clear the sensory field and focus the mind internally. Visualization may be of a helpful color, a geometrical design (like a yantra), an image in the world of nature, or a deity or guru (as per the person's natural inclination).

4. Repeat an affirmation to increase positive thought power, like calling up your soul's inherent freedom from pain, unhappiness and bondage. Or perform some prayer for healing or inner growth.

5. Repeat a mantra to calm the subconscious mind. Mantras should be done at least 108 times before meditation as well as periodically during the day, particularly when the mind is not occupied.

6. Silently observe the mind and let it empty itself out. The meditator should take the role of a witness and learn to look at the contents of the mind, just like watching the waves and debris flow down a rapidly moving stream.

7. Meditation proper, which can be either knowledge-oriented or devotion-oriented depending upon one's temperament, trying to contact God or the higher Self through the natural movement of the heart.

Specific Meditational Approaches

Once one has understood the general approach of meditation, one can focus on a particular meditational approach most suitable to one's aspiration.

Devotional Meditation

Devotional meditation depends upon a form of God, avatar

or great teacher to worship, or a relationship with the divine as father, mother, teacher, or beloved. This is largely a personal matter and may be conditioned by one's religious background, so it is generally not something for the ayurvedic therapist to decide. Human beings should worship the divine in whatever form appeals to their inmost heart. Anything less is spiritual tyranny.

Hindu deities have specific ayurvedic correspondences. For example, Ganesh, the elephant-headed god and remover of obstacles, can be used to increase kapha and ojas. Hanuman, who has the form of a monkey and is born of the Wind, promotes prana and controls vata. Skanda, the divine child, warrior and son of fire, develops tejas.

The Goddess Kali, who controls death and destruction, can be used to increase prana, control vata, and remove life-threatening diseases. The God Shiva, who rules over the subconscious and the superconscious, helps us overcome fear, anxiety and trauma. The avatar Rama protects children from harm. There are dozens of such examples.

Another important form of devotional worship is the planetary deities, the cosmic powers behind the forces of time and karma. This is done from the standpoint of Vedic astrology. Deities of fiery planets like the Sun, Mars and Ketu (south lunar node) are good for increasing pitta, tejas and agni. Deities of watery planets like the Moon, Venus and Jupiter are good for increasing kapha, ojas and the dhatus. Deities of airy planets like Saturn, Mercury and Rahu (north lunar node) are good for increasing prana and vata.

Knowledge Meditation

Knowledge-oriented meditation aims at spiritual knowledge, which is self-knowledge. It is of two types, passive and active. Passive meditation involves taking the attitude of a witness and observing one's thoughts. Or it may consist of holding to a state of receptivity, opening up to the divine presence or the void. Passive meditation generally begins with external objects, like a ghee lamp or something in nature like a tree or clouds in the sky, then focuses gradually inward on the body, senses, prana, emotions, thought, ego and ultimately the higher Self or the silent divine beyond all concepts.

Active meditation involves some form of inquiry like "Who am I?" or seeking one's true nature. This involves tracing the I-thought back to its origin in pure consciousness. It has been explained in the works of Ramana Maharshi and other teachers of Advaita Vedanta, as well as in traditional Advaitic texts like the *Yoga Vasishta* or the works of Shankaracharya. It requires seeking the Self behind the body, breath, senses, mind or whatever we are observing. It is an extension of ayurvedic counseling techniques, helping us understand the workings of the body and mind.

General Considerations for Meditation

Meditation Room

One should have a special room for meditation, containing an altar, special pictures or holy books, and decorated so as to have a spiritual energy. The room should be well ventilated and have natural light. An office or study room can be used if necessary but not a bedroom or a basement.

Meditation Seat

One should have a comfortable seat or chair for meditation. A meditation rug or cushion made of wool or silk is helpful. For meditation, one should sit facing east or north. One can sprinkle a little water around the seat along with reciting a simple mantra like OM before one meditates to purify the seat.

Meditation Ritual

Perform a short ritual before meditation like offering a fragrant oil (for the earth element), water (for the water element), a ghee lamp or candle (for the fire element), incense (for the air element), and a flower (for the ether element). These can be placed before a statue or picture of a deity or guru or simply offered to the divine in whatever way one wishes. Such a ritual cleanses the psychic air and prepares the room for meditation. One can also ring a bell or do some chant or prayer.

Mala/ Meditation Beads

A *mala* or rosary should be used for counting mantras. Rudraksha is good for increasing tejas and for worship of Lord Shiva. Crystal is good for worshipping the Goddess. Tulsi beads are specific for Lord Vishnu (Rama and Krishna). For repeating bija mantras (single-syllable mantras), one can count off eight or sixteen mantras per bead to make the counting easier. Mantras may require over one hundred thousand repetitions for them to gain real power. They must be embedded into the subconscious mind to become really effective.

Longer Mantras

There are many longer mantras or prayers that have powerful healing properties. Mahamrityunjaya mantra to Rudra-Shiva is good for protection against injuries and febrile disease. Gayatri mantra to the sun increases vital energy and strengthens the heart. This is mentioned for the sake of those who know these mantras or who receive them as part of their training. Various spiritual traditions have prayers or hymns that can be used in similar ways.

Time for Meditation

Meditation should be done on a regular daily basis, just

like eating or sleeping. Yet certain days are more favorable. Thursday, the day of Jupiter, is the best day for meditation, followed by Wednesday (Mercury), Monday (Moon) and Friday (Venus). Meditation is also better during the waxing moon. One can consult a Vedic astrologer for favorable times for meditation both during the year and according to the periods of one's life, particularly if one wants to begin intense meditational practices.

The best time of the day for meditation is early morning before dawn, the hour of Brahman. Sunrise and sunset are other good periods. Many people find sunset to be the best because by that time of the day the main work is done and one can look within. These are mainly vata times, in which vata and its related systems like the mind and prana can be more easily worked upon. Immediately before sleep is another important time to clear the mind.

Meditation in the morning should be followed by physical exercise like yoga asanas, walking or mild aerobic exercises. Then tea and a light meal can be taken. However, if a person has a lot of ama (toxins) or kapha in the system, or a lot of mucus, as in the case of sinus allergies, then exercise and pranayama may be necessary first to dispel the inertia. Otherwise the mind and brain may be too dull or congested for meditation. Vatas may feel too tired to get up early for meditation. In this case they should try to compensate by going to bed earlier and taking a nap in the afternoon. Pittas like to be night people but can discipline themselves to arise earlier if they make the effort. For people who have trouble staying awake during morning meditation, a morning walk can be helpful first or a walking meditation instead of a sitting meditation.

In the evening, meditation should be followed by sleep, so that a deep sleep can ensue. In the evening there should be no sensory distraction, like television, immediately before meditation or after it. One should avoid disturbing the mind after evening meditation or one will lose much of the benefit of the practice. Meditation should not be done immediately after eating, particularly after a heavy meal.

Duration of Meditation

Meditation should consist of about fifteen minutes of pranayama, fifteen minutes of mantra, and then fifteen minutes of silent or devotional meditation as a minimum. It should be done at least twice a day, morning and evening. After one has mastered this as a continual practice, the length of meditation can be increased and it can be done three times a day or more.

The most important thing is consistency of practice. It is better to meditate a little every day than to do a lot of meditation on an irregular basis. Occasional meditation intensives or retreats are helpful but should be followed up by consistent daily practice.

Ayurvedic Meditations

Ayurvedic doctors often perform a meditation upon Lord Dhanvantari before treatment or before classes. One can use the mantra:

> Om Dham Dhanvantaraye Namah!

Others do a meditation on Lord Ganesha, which removes all obstacles for treatment, using his mantra:

> Om Gam Ganeshaya Namah!

One can also meditate upon one's *ishta devata* or chosen form of God to worship.

Ayurvedic practitioners often perform prayers or mantras in the presence of the patient as part of the treatment. The patients may be encouraged to join in the process. In addition it is best for practitioners to do some silent meditation before seeing clients to bring a positive healing energy into the clinic or treatment room.

MEDITATION ACCORDING TO DOSHIC TYPES

Vata Types

Meditation

Vata types should practice meditation in order to calm their restless minds and nerves and to relieve their inherent tendency to fear and anxiety. Meditation can take them very far in overcoming their main problem in life — a hypersensitive and hyperactive mind and vital force. Meditation helps them sleep, alleviates their nervous digestion, and strengthens their immune system, which are their main areas of weakness.

However, vatas must be careful because meditation done wrongly can be ungrounding and quickly spaces them out. They can get lost in their thoughts or their prana can become disturbed. For this reason, vatas should first learn the art of concentration so that their minds do not wander. It is better for them to do mantra or visualization rather than try to empty their minds, which may already have too much of the ether element within them.

Yet vata types should not try to stop or suppress their natural mental activity either. They should let their minds move freely and naturally while seeking the deeper truth of life. They must learn to harness their abundant mental energy for meditation, which for them should be like the flight of an eagle. They must let their mind soar without losing its focus.

Asana and Pranayama

Vata people should first make sure that they are sitting comfortably and that their body and joints are at ease. They should do some relaxation exercises to release tension before sitting, or talk a walk first. Vata people have trouble sitting still and without some asana practice may not last long in the same posture.

Vatas suffer from low energy that weakens concentration. They should deepen their breath so that they have sufficient prana for meditation. Pranayama may initially make vatas feel tired because it reduces the hyperactivity of vata. If this occurs they should do a little rapid or vigorous deep breathing until their mental clarity returns. Yet vatas should never be forceful with pranayama and should introduce it gradually.

Visualization, Affirmation and Mantra

For visualization, vata people should use earthy, watery and fiery images like a mountain, a lake or the ocean, flowers like a lotus or rose, light like the fire or the sun at dawn. Anti-vata color therapy can be used, like the colors gold or saffron. This they should do for a few minutes to clear their mental field.

Vatas should affirm the basic peace and fearlessness of their higher nature and learn to let go of worry and anxiety. They should have faith in some form of God or great teacher to take care of them on the inner planes. They should call upon the protection of the forms of God and the Goddess and the gurus to help them with problems that they cannot solve of their own accord.

Anti-vata mantras are best, like RAM, SHRIM, or HRIM. Vatas should repeat such mantras during the meditation period and also do them during the day, particularly when vata appears to be getting out of balance. Often it is better if these mantras are muttered in a low voice, which keeps vata types energized but calm.

Devotional Meditation

Vata types require benefic forms of divine energy, particularly forms of the divine Father and Mother, the parental relationship that is calming, supporting and nourishing. Protective forms of the Divine Mother like Durga and Tara are especially good. Benefic forms of the Divine Father like Shiva as the Lord of Yogis or Vishnu as the avatar and savior Rama are similarly very helpful. Ganesh can be very grounding. Hanuman in particular gives the power of prana and represents higher vata characteristics.

Knowledge Meditation

Vata people should meditate upon the eternal and immutable nature of truth in order to slow down their thoughts. They require contact with dharma or universal law in order to give support to their restless minds. They must learn to contact the changeless and immortal Self within the heart or the still and silent expanse of pure Being. Vatas need to become stabilized in their inner nature and not worry about the fluctuations of the external world. They must turn within and forget the world, its disturbances and its distractions.

Pitta Types

Meditation

Pitta people need to meditate in order to release their anger and aggression and let go of their generally willful and controlling approach to life. Pittas usually have good concentration and can meditate more easily than other types. Mantra and meditation can be a good way for them to focus their strong mental energy in a positive manner, directing their attention toward an inner goal.

Pittas should be careful to meditate peacefully and not try to turn meditation into another form of achievement or conquest. For them meditation can become too focused and even narrow-minded, an attempt to control rather than a release of tension. They must learn to expand their mind and heart in meditation, using their inherent light to reveal the truth. Meditation should leave them feeling cool and calm in mind and heart, like gentle waves moving across a lake in the moonlight.

Asana and Pranayama

Pitta people should first make sure to be cool and relaxed in their meditation posture. They should not do any strenuous exercise before meditation or work up a sweat. They should do pranayama that is cooling, emphasizing lunar breathing or breathing through the left nostril. Shitali can also be done. They should release their internal heat through the breath before meditation.

Visualization, Affirmation and Mantra

Pittas should visualize non-fiery images like a mountain forest, a lake or the ocean, rain clouds, the deep blue sky, flowers with cooling colors, the moon or the stars. Anti-pitta color therapy can be used, like the colors white, dark blue or emerald green.

Pitta people should do affirmations increasing forgiveness, compassion and love and surrendering anger. They should do prayers of peace and happiness for all beings. They should also seek forgiveness for the wrong or forceful actions they have done that might have harmed other creatures.

Anti-pitta mantras are indicated like SHAM, SHRIM, or OM. These should be repeated silently. They should also be used when pitta emotions like anger get elevated during the day, repeated in a slow and relaxed manner.

Devotional Meditation

Pittas should meditate upon cooling and calming forms of the Divine Father and Mother. Forms of the Goddess — including Lakshmi born of the ocean, and Uma-Parvati, Shiva's wife and the daughter of the snow mountain — can be helpful.

Forms of the God include Vishnu and Shiva in their benefic forms of water and space. While pittas may incline to more fiery or wrathful forms, they should be careful with them as this may increase their fire.

Meditating upon God as the divine friend or divine beloved is another way. Pittas can transform their passion into devotion but should keep that devotion receptive and peaceful. They can take the attitude of a warrior for the divine but must be cautious not to use this as a way of promoting more aggressive energy.

Knowledge Meditation

Pitta types can be very critical in their minds, caught in their own opinions and judgments that prevents them from getting beyond the field of thought. They should use this as power to inquire into the nature of consciousness and contact the higher Self beyond the mind, developing the art of discrimination.

Pittas benefit from meditating upon infinite space beyond all the limitations of the critical mind. If they can direct their concentration in a beneficial way they can discover the light within the heart, which is like the moon and is beyond the heat and agitation of the outer mind. Silence and receptivity of mind and heart aid in this process.

Kapha Types

Meditation

Kapha types require meditation in order to let go of emotional attachment and to counter mental stagnation and lethargy. Meditation helps them release possessiveness and heaviness into the space of consciousness, in which alone is true happiness and abundance. Kaphas may require encouragement, stimulation or motivation to get them into meditation and often do better meditating in a group. For them a more disciplined approach to meditation is required, even if it does not seem immediately to be having much result.

Kaphas are likely to fall asleep during meditation. For this reason they should do more active forms of meditation, including mantra and pranayama, or combine meditation with activity. They are also prone to fall into their imagination or daydream. They need to cultivate a wakeful attention to counter the inherent lassitude of their minds.

Asana and Pranayama

Kapha people should first do some physical exercise to open their circulation and dispel stagnation before taking a seating posture. This may require some mild aerobic exercise but not too strenuous as to disturb the mind. Walking meditation is good for them.

They should also do some vigorous pranayama, emphasizing quick inhalation and exhalation (like bhastrika), or right nostril breathing to move their energy. Then they can proceed with a more calm type of pranayama. They should combine meditation with periods of pranayama to keep their energy moving.

Visualization, Affirmation and Mantra

Kapha people should focus on images which increase the fire, air and ether elements, like the sun, the wind moving through the trees, or the expanse of clear blue sky. Anti-kapha color therapy can also be used, like gold, blue and orange.

Kapha people need to affirm the detachment of their higher nature. Such affirmations like "In my true Self I am independent, free and of the nature of space" are useful for them. They should also seek to develop their kapha energy of love by directing thoughts of love and care for all creatures.

They should do stimulating and clearing mantras, first out loud for a few minutes, then repeating them with the breath. Such mantras are OM, HUM or AIM.

Devotional Meditation

Kaphas are highly loving people and benefit by cultivating a devotional relationship with the divine. Faith and surrender are usually easy for them. They are open to many forms of devotional worship. Loving forms of the divine are most attractive to them. However, they may require more stimulating or wrathful forms of the God and Goddess to motivate them, like the wrathful forms of Shiva or the form of Kali.

Kaphas should avoid getting caught in excessive emotionality; devotion should not become a form of self-indulgence. This requires purity of heart and mind, using devotion to reduce attachment, release emotion, and lighten the human personality and ego. They should also avoid getting attached to the outer forms of devotion. They must learn to contact the infinite and formless through the forms that they use.

Knowledge Meditation

Kapha people need to learn the formlessness and infinity of reality in order to release their attachment to form and limitation. They are particularly good at meditating upon the eternal, immutable aspect of truth. They can cultivate unchanging peace as the basis of the mental field.

Meditation upon the void is particularly good for them because it increases space in the mind. It can be combined with meditation upon the inner light, bringing more fire into their minds. Inquiry forms of meditation may be hard for them because their minds like to rest in a comfortable state. This is not always good, however, as they can confuse such a contented state of mind with higher truth. Kaphas must learn to rouse their attention to always go further. They should not rest content until they have gone beyond their personal limitations. They should view meditation like climbing a series of mountain peaks along a great journey, not stopping along the way, no matter how pleasant.

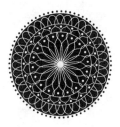

Ayurveda and yoga culminate in the art of meditation. The ayurvedic knowledge of the doshas and pranas helps us use meditation for healing and balancing purposes. The yogic knowledge of the mind and the gunas helps us use meditation for Self-realization. Meditation is like the pinnacle of the pyramid of Vedic knowledge. It culminates in a sharp point that penetrates into the infinite, but it rests on a broad base that goes deep into the Earth.

May this wisdom help you in all aspects of your life and consciousness!

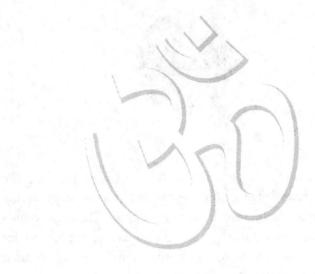

APPENDIX 1

The Vedic Connection

The *Vedas* are the great mantric scriptures set forth by Himalayan rishis, yogis and sages who lived many thousands of years ago at the reputed beginning of this World Age or *yuga*, at the dawn of human history. They are said to manifest the wisdom of the cosmic mind that is the origin and support of the universe and the foundation of natural law. The four *Vedas* were passed down through long oral and written traditions dating from before the time of Krishna, four or five thousand years ago.[41]

The *Vedas* present the broader system of Self and cosmic knowledge of which yoga and Ayurveda are specific manifestations. Both Ayurveda and yoga arose as Vedic schools, taught by lineages of Vedic seers, projecting Vedic knowledge into specific practical forms. Both look back upon Vedic texts for their authority. They follow the Vedic vision into their respective fields of health and spiritual practice.

The *Vedas*

The *Vedas* are primarily three in number and each relates to an important practice of yoga and Ayurveda. The three *Vedas* reflect a mantric approach that comprehends all aspects of life. They set forth the Vedic ritual, *yajna* or fire sacrifice, which mirrors the process of cosmic creation. Inwardly it is a yoga practice balancing agni and soma (fire and water), the perceiver and the perceived within us. This general Vedic yajna uncovers all the powers of the universe and can be used to realize all the goals of life from health to liberation. A fourth Veda, the *Atharva Veda*, provides mantras for specific topics, including personal matters, and similarly covers all aspects of life.

CORRESPONDENCES OF THE THREE *VEDAS*

Rig Veda	Yajur Veda	Sama Veda
Divine Speech	Divine Prana	Divine Mind
Mantra Yoga	Prana Yoga	Dhyana Yoga
knowledge	practice	Realization
waking state	dream state	deep sleep
Earth	Atmosphere	Heaven
Fire (Agni)	Wind (Vayu)	Sun (Surya)

The Vedic yajna is a healing process aimed at restoring to wholeness the divine consciousness that has entered into us and become fragmented through the mind, body and senses. The purpose of the Vedic yajna is to heal or put back together the purusha or cosmic being that has sacrificed itself to become the world. This reintegration of the Creator and creation, or God and the soul, is the foundation of yoga as well, which means union. Ayurveda arises out of this Vedic urge not merely for personal healing but for healing the divine consciousness that has fallen into the material world.

The existent Vedic texts are vehicles of a deeper cosmic wisdom that is woven into all aspects of life. In this regard the *Vedas* are infinite and eternal. They are inherent in the cosmic Mind and manifest along with every cycle of creation as the vibrations of the divine Word through which the universe comes into being. Our soul and its creative forces work through a portion of this power.

The Vedic mantras reflect the energy of life. They are said to be inherent in prana, which is not only the life-force but the entire movement of cosmic energy. As vehicles for the cosmic prana, the *Vedas* possess tremendous vitality and healing power. Prana itself creates language, as speech itself arises from the breath. This creative word holds the seed or archetypal forms of creation that the *Vedas* portray. Through the *Vedas*, therefore, we gain access to the very powers of creation that can change nature itself.

There are two main parts of the *Vedas*. First is the mantra portion (*Samhita*), which is the foundation just discussed. Second is the commentary portion, which itself consists of three parts — the *Brahmanas, Aranyakas* and *Upanishads* — making up a total of four sections. The *Brahmanas* deal with the details of various rituals, both external and internal (yogic), individual and collective. The *Aranyakas* are similar but have a more internal nature, providing themes for meditation and ascetic practices The *Upanishads* are predominantly philosophical in nature and provide a summary of Vedic insights and knowledge. Yet the distinction between *Brahmanas* and *Upanishads* is only a matter of degree. The *Brahmanas* teach much spiritual wisdom or Self-knowledge and the *Upanishads* present rituals and practices of various types. The *Upanishads* are the basis of Vedanta, yoga and the later spiritual and philosophical disciplines that derive from the *Vedas*.

The Six Schools of Vedic Insight

Out of the *Vedas* arose six schools of philosophy, *shad darshanas*, which literally means six ways of seeing or insight. These were designed to show the logical, metaphysical and cosmological implications with the Vedic mantras. Classical yoga as expounded by Patanjali in the *Yoga Sutras* is one of these six schools of Vedic philosophy. Patanjali himself was said to be in the line of the great yogi and Vedic sage Yajnavalkya, one of the seers of the *Yajur Veda* and *Brihadaranyaka Upanishad,* and Patanjali was said to be a teacher of the *Sama Veda* as well. Hiranyagarbha, a name for the sun god as the cosmic Creator, was the traditional founder of the Yoga system.

The Six Schools of Vedic Philosophy and Their Founders:

1. *Nyaya* — Logic School — Gautama

2. *Vaisheshika* — Atomic School — Kannada

3. *Samkhya* — Cosmic Principle School — Kapila

4. *Yoga* — Yoga School — Hiranyagarbha

5. *Purva Mimamsa* — Ritualistic School — Jaimini

6. *Uttara Mimamsa/*Vedanta — Theological or Metaphysical School — Badarayana

Nyaya and Vaisheshika are schools of logical philosophy, similar to the system of Plato in Western thought. All Vedic schools, including Ayurveda and yoga, insist upon the development of strong rational skills, which comes about through training in Nyaya-Vaisheshika. Both the yogi and the ayurvedic doctor must support their conclusions with the proper logic, though this is made subordinate to a higher intuitive perception.

Samkhya provides the background philosophy and cosmology both for yoga and Ayurveda, as already noted earlier in the book. It has a scientific view, examining both internal and external reality. The Samkhya system outlines the tattvas or cosmic principles that yogic practice seeks to realize.

However, there is a slight difference between Samkhya and yoga. Samkhya is more concerned with knowledge of the tattvas (soul, mind, sense organs, motor organs, elements), while yoga is concerned more with purification of the corresponding tattvas within us. Yoga prepares us for the knowledge of Samkhya because only when a tattva is purified can we understand it. Yoga adds a theistic view to Samkhya and could be called a theistic form of Samkhya. Yet the approach of yoga is more practical and so more of a technology than a philosophy and can be used with various philosophical systems.

Yoga occurs along with Samkhya as a common term in late Vedic texts, like the *Bhagavad Gita* of Sri Krishna, which is also said to be a yogic scripture. Yoga is commonly mentioned in the *Upanishads*, particularly the *Prashna, Katha* and *Svestasvatara*. References to Yoga can be found in all the *Vedas* going back to the *Rig Veda* itself.[42] Many great modern yogis like Sri Aurobindo, Ganapati Muni or Paramahamsa Yogananda have explained the Vedic basis of yoga.

The ritualistic school, Purva Mimamsa, emphasizes proper performance of rituals for both individual and social welfare, using special prayers and offerings to link us with the beneficent forces of the universe. These rituals are good for purifying body and mind and prepare us for meditation. This is the field of karma yoga or the yoga of service.

The term Vedanta is used specifically for the Uttara Mimamsa school, which is the most concerned of the six systems with the proper interpretation of Vedic texts (though all the six systems share this concern). Vedanta or the theological/metaphysical school discusses the nature of God, the soul, the Absolute and their relationship. There are several schools of Vedanta, which became in time the most important and extensive of the Vedic philosophical traditions.

Non-dualistic (*advaita*) Vedanta, taught by the great philosopher Shankara (seventh century), makes both God and the soul to be manifestations of the Absolute, which constitutes their real Self. It emphasizes jnana yoga or the yoga of knowledge, such as made popular today through the teachings of the modern sage of South India, Ramana Maharshi.

Dualistic (*dvaita*) Vedanta, like that taught by Madhva (fourteenth century), makes God and the soul to be different but eternally related. It teaches devotion to God and the subordination of the soul to His grace. It emphasizes bhakti yoga or the yoga of devotion. Many Vaishnavas (worshippers of Vishnu) follow this line, including the Krishna movement of Prabhupada.

An intermediate school, the qualified non-dualist Visishtadvaita school of Ramanuja (twelfth century), is also important. It is devotional and Vaishnava in nature like the dualistic school. It has a special connection to yoga. Krishnamacharya of Madras is the guru of many yoga teachers famous in the West, such as B.K.S. Iyengar, Pattabhi Jois or T.V. Deshikar, who was of this line.

Yoga is closely aligned with Vedanta of some sort. Most of the original yoga teachers who came to the West — Swami Vivekananda, Rama Tirtha, Paramahamsa Yogananda, Swami Rama, or the many disciples of Swami Shivananda — taught Yoga-Vedanta of the advaitic line. Most ayurvedic teachers are also Vedantins.

Vedanta is close to Samkhya, and in later India took over much of the place of Samkhya, whose main teachings it adapted. Samkhya itself was originally a Vedic system, with its own commentaries on Vedantic texts. Yet there is a slight difference between Vedanta, Samkhya and Yoga.

Samkhya and Vedanta are both concerned with knowledge of the tattvas. However, Samkhya is concerned with knowledge of all the tattvas leading to the purusha or individual soul. Vedanta, particularly in the advaitic school, is aimed mainly at paramatman (the supreme soul) and Brahman (the absolute), the highest tattva, and has less concern with the lower tattvas. Devotional Vedantic schools are theological in nature and concerned mainly with Ishvara tattva or the Creator, which is not a separate tattva in classical Samkhya.

To use Sanskrit terms: Samkhya is concerned with *tattva vichara* or inquiry into the nature of the tattvas. Advaita Vedanta involves *Atma tattva vichara*, inquiry into the Self or the highest tattva. Dualistic Vedanta's main concern is *Ishvara tattva vichara*, inquiry into the nature of God and our relationship with Him (or Her, as the divine is not limited to the masculine gender in Hindu thought).

Yoga is concerned with *tattva shuddhi*, which means not only purification of the tattvas but research into them. Yoga, in purifying the tattvas, allows for inquiry into them to proceed, which cannot occur when mind and body are in an impure condition. The proper practice of yoga in all of its eight limbs up to samadhi, therefore, provides us the aptitude to pursue Samkhya and Vedanta. For this reason many Vedantins require that their students first gain proficiency in yoga so that they have the right training to proceed on their knowledge quest.

Yet yoga in some form is part of all six schools, which are integral parts of the same Vedic *darshana* or way of seeing. Yoga provides the practical foundation for the insights that the other systems seek to develop — preparing body, prana and mind to become tools of inner inquiry. In this regard yoga is probably the most universal of the six systems and is the main link between them. Ayurveda provides the foundation of right living for yoga and for all the six systems, whose world view and practices it shares, so it also is common to all the six systems.

Yoga and Ayurveda, at least to some degree, were adopted by non-Vedic systems in India as well. Buddhist, Jain and even Sufi teachers have used various insights and methods of Ayurveda and yoga. Many connections are through tantra, which employs aspects of yoga and Ayurveda and has Hindu and Buddhist forms. Tibetan medicine, for example, is predominantly ayurvedic.

Ayurveda and Vedas/Upavedas

The Upavedas supplement the Vedas with more specific applications of Vedic teachings into the cultural field. Ayurveda arose as a secondary Veda or Upaveda generally connected with the *Atharva Veda*. This is because the *Atharva Veda* first presents specific mantras and methods for treating various diseases. However, Ayurveda is connected with the other Vedas, which are all concerned with self-knowledge and internal integration. It has a close connection with *Yajur Veda* which describes the Vedic ritual aimed at healing both the Cosmic Being and the individual soul.[43]

The Upavedas are:

1. Ayurveda — healing arts
2. Dhanur Veda — martial arts
3. Sthapatya Veda — architecture, sculpture and geomancy
4. Gandharva Veda — music, poetry and dance

Ayurveda is closely connected with all the Upavedas. It relies upon Dhanur Veda or the martial arts for exercise recommendations and styles of massage and body work, particularly the treatment of the *marmas* or sensitive points on the body. The marmas are mainly described in Dhanur Veda. Many yoga asanas also reflect the insights of Dhanur Veda.

Ayurveda employs Gandharva Veda for its subtle therapies of music and art, which are very important in healing both mind and body. Yogas of music and sound develop out of Gandharva Veda.

Sthapatya Veda, more commonly called *Vastu*, shows the right design of structures to bring in wholesome earth and spatial energies. This is essential for the proper orientation and construction of clinics, hospitals, and healing rooms. Some people may suffer from disease mainly due to the fact that the wrong construction of their houses exposes them to harmful directional forces. For this reason, many ayurvedic doctors will question patients on how their house is situated as part of their diagnosis. Yoga uses Vastu for the orientation of temples, ashrams and meditation rooms. For example, the yogic recommendation to meditate facing east or north reflects the considerations of Vastu.

The Vedangas/Vedic Astrology

There are six *Vedangas* or limbs of the *Vedas*. These are closer to the *Vedas* than the Upavedas, being part of the *Vedas* themselves, the main tools used to interpret them.

1. *Jyotish* — astrology
2. *Kalpa* — rules of ritual
3. *Shiksha* — pronunciation
4. *Vyakarana* — grammar
5. *Nirukta* — etymology
6. *Chhandas* — meters

Of the six vedangas, jyotish or Vedic astrology is the most important. For Ayurveda it helps determine the basic health potential of the person, their disease tendency and possibility of recovery. This is particularly important for patients suffering from severe illnesses and for illnesses that are not responding to normal treatment measures. Vedic astrology is also used for the timing of treatment and for preparing medicines. Even the right therapy done at the wrong time may not bring good results. Astrology helps us understand psychological problems, which are often evident from the birth chart. It is useful in ayurvedic therapies, particularly for showing what gems are best for a person to wear.

Vedic astrology is helpful in yoga for determining individual spiritual potential, for the timing of yogic practices and, particularly, for mantra initiation. An examination of the birth chart is important either for ayurvedic or yogic concerns and is an integral part of a Vedic approach to life. For this reason many ayurvedic and yoga practitioners study jyotish or at least make sure to have access to a good astrologer to consult with as needed.

Four of the six vedangas deal with language. They are the basis of the Sanskrit language and its precise terminology for both yoga and Ayurveda. They are part of the path of mantra yoga, which is very important in both yoga and Ayurveda. Ayurveda uses mantra as the main tool for healing the mind. Yoga uses it as the main tool for purifying the mind and unfolding its inner powers and faculties. Mantra is the most important tool of yoga, Ayurveda and jyotish and the foundation of Vedic science.

In summary, yoga arose as the application of Vedic wisdom for Self-realization. Ayurveda arose as a Vedic method for healing and right living. Both systems are best understood in a Vedic context and help us understand the principles of Vedic living.[44] Yoga provides the means for purification of the mind (chitta-shuddhi) to enable us to gain Self-realization through Vedanta (Self-knowledge). Ayurveda affords us purification of the body (deha-shuddhi) for optimal health and energy. Vastu gives us purification of the home (griha-shanti) for right orientation in space. Jyotish gives us purification from negative planetary influences (graha-shanti) for right orientation in time.

Putting together this entire system of Vedic knowledge — combining Ayurveda, yoga and related disciplines — we have a tremendous resource that can transform both ourselves and our planet if we apply it in our daily lives. This is one of the keys to higher evolution in humanity, a subject that requires much more attention in this age of crisis and transition.

APPENDIX 2

Endnotes

1 Note Appendix, The Vedic Connection.

2 For example, the study of the *Yoga Sutras* of Patanjali is usually combined with that of the *Samkhya Karika* of Ishvara Krishna.

3 This idea of Prana Purusha or Prana Atman is common in the *Upanishads*, note *Brihadaranyaka* I.6.3 for example.

4 Purusha visesha of *Yoga Sutras* I.23.

5 *Yoga Sutras* I.18.

6 The yoga system introduces a fourth aspect of the mind called *Chitta*. This is used for the general mental field as a whole, of which Buddhi, Ahamkara and Manas are functions. It can be identified with our mental Prakriti, though some thinkers place it in the field of the Buddhi, and others in the field of Manas.

7 The *Vedas* speak about how Vayu or the cosmic air principle arises from the Sun.

8 *Brihat Yogi Yajnavalkya Smriti* 9.5: "Vayu and Agni dwelling in the heart are called God and the soul."

9 *Yoga Sutras* I.2.

10 *Yoga Sutras* I.3.

11 *Yoga Sutras* II. 1-2.

12 *Yoga Sutras* II.1.1.

13 This is called Pancha Kosha Yoga and Pancha Kosha Ayurveda

14 The *Vedas* call it Hiranyagarbha or the golden fetus, from which is born the Divine Sun of enlightenment. It is also called the golden sheath (hiranmaya kosha) within the heart.

15 Called Linga in Sanskrit.

16 Note *The Holy Science* of Swami Sri Yukteswar, Sutra 14, p. 35.

17 I have examined the issue of Prana, Tejas and Ojas in more detail in my book *Tantric Yoga and the Wisdom Goddesses* pp. 183-219.

18 See also *Brahmacharya* by Swami Shivananda.

19 Sanskrit - amritopastaranam asi svaha

20 Sanskrit - amritapidhanam asi svaha

21 Note the *Bhagavad Gita* IV. 25-33 for an explication of the various Yajnas or fire offerings,

including those of different yogic practices.

22 *Maitrayani Upanishad* VI.1-5

23 *Satapatha Brahmana* VIII.4.7

24 *Satapatha Brahmana* X.1.4.1-7

25 *Prashna Upanishad* III. 9-10

26 Note my discussion of the Chakras in *Tantric Yoga and the Wisdom Goddesses*, Part III. Chapters 1 and 2.

27 Note Vyasa's commentary on *Yoga Sutras I.12* which describes the Chitta Nadi and its outward flow relating to the senses and its inward flow relating to discrimination.

28 Note Bibliography for Ayurvedic cookbooks, particularly those of Amadea Morningstar, who also has a book on Ayurvedic Cooking for Westerners. Note the work of Maya Tiwari for a more in-depth examination of the spiritual aspects of ayurvedic diet.

29 Note *Yoga of Herbs* in this regard.

30 *Susruta Samhita Chiktisa Sthanam* 29 and 30.4.

31 *Atharva Veda* XI.6.15.

32 *Atharva Veda* XIX.39.5.

33 Please examine *Ayurveda and the Mind* for more information on this fascinating topic. Note bibliography.

34 For more information please examine *Ayurveda and Pancha Karma* by Dr. Sunil Joshi.

35 That is why the *Yoga Sutras* II.47 emphasizes relaxation of effort and moving the mind into the infinite through Asana.

36 *Maitriyani Upanishad* VI.1.

37 *Shatapatha Brahmana* X.1.4.12.

38 *Charaka Samhita Sarira Sthana* I.128.

39 "That which is the vibration of Prana Vayu (Prana spanda) is also the vibration of the mind (Chitta spanda);" *Laghu Yoga Vasishta* V.10.25.

40 I have discussed the levels of the mind and their general Doshic connections, in *Ayurveda and the Mind*.

41 For more information on this topic note, *In Search of the Cradle of Civilization* (Feuerstein, Frawley and Kak) and *Gods, Sages and Kings: Vedic Secrets of Ancient Civilization* (Frawley).

42 For example, *Rig Veda* V.81.1 or I.18.7.

43 "The Gods made the sacrifice (Yajna) as the medicine." *Shukla Yajur Veda* XIX.1

44 For a study of Vedic deities examine *Wisdom of the Ancient Seers* (Frawley) or *Secret of the Veda* (Sri Aurobindo).

APPENDIX 3

Sanskrit Glossary

Agni — fire as a cosmic principle

Ahamkara — ego or sense of separate self

Ahimsa — non-violence or non-harming

Ananda — bliss or divine love

Anandamaya Kosha — sheath of bliss, heart or deeper feeling nature

Anna — food or nourishment as a cosmic principle

Annamaya Kosha — sheath of food or physical body

Antahkarana — internal instrument, mind on all levels

Apana — downward-moving prana

Asanas — yogic postures

Astral Body — subtle body of pure impressions and prana

Astral Plane — subtle world of pure impressions, dream plane

Atman — true Self, sense of pure I am

Ayurveda — yogic science of healing

Bandha — yogic locks

Basti — ayurvedic enemas

Bhakti Yoga — yoga of devotion

Bija Mantra — single syllable mantras like OM

Brahman — Absolute Reality

Buddhi — intelligence

Causal Body — body of samskaras, gunas, or deepest tendencies, field of the soul

Causal Plane — source world of creation, realm of the ideal deep sleep plane

Chakras — energy centers of subtle body

Chitta — a general term for the mind on all levels, including the subconscious; a specific term for the deepest level of the mind or bliss sheath

Devi — the Goddess
Dharana — concentration
Dharma — the law of our nature, truth principle
Dhyana — meditation

Ganesha - deity of knowledge and protection
Gunas — three prime qualities of Nature of sattva, rajas and tamas
Guru — spiritual guide
Hanuman — deity of prana and devotion
Hatha Yoga — yoga of asana, pranayama and meditation, effort oriented
Homa — Vedic fire offerings

Ida — left nostril or lunar nadi
Indra — Vedic deity of prana and energy
Ishvara — God or the Creator
Ishvari — Divine Mother, feminine aspect of God
Jiva — individual soul
Jnana Yoga — yoga of Self-knowledge

Kali — goddess of energy and transformation
Kapha — biological water humor
Karma — effect of our past actions, including from previous births
Karma Yoga — yoga of ritual, work and service
Kosha — body, sheath or encasement for the soul
Kundalini — latent energy of spiritual development

Lakshmi — goddess of beauty and divine grace
Laya Yoga — yoga of mergence in the divine sound current
Mahat — Divine Mind or Cosmic Intelligence
Manas — outer or sensory aspect of mind
Manomaya Kosha — sheath of impressions or outer mind

Mantra — seed sounds used for healing or yogic purposes
Marmas — sensitive points on the body

Nadis — channel systems of subtle body
Nasya — ayurvedic nasal treatments
Neti Pot — small pot for pouring salt water through the nostrils
Niyamas — yogic disciplines and principles of personal behavior
Ojas — vital essence of kapha

Pancha Karma — ayurvedic detoxification procedure
Pingala — right nostril or solar nadi
Pitta — biological fire humor
Prakriti — nature
Prana — vital force, breath
Pranamaya Kosha — sheath of prana or vital energy
Pranayama — control or expansion of vital force
Prarthana — prayer or seeking of blessings
Pratyahara — control or introversion of the mind and senses
Puja — Hindu rituals
Purusha — inner spirit, Self

Raja Yoga — Integral Yoga system of Patanjali in *Yoga Sutras*
Rajas — quality of action and agitation
Rajasic — of the nature of rajas

Samadhi — absorption
Samana — balancing vital force
Samkalpa — will, intention, resolution
Samkhya — philosophy of the 24 tattvas
Samskaras — deep-seated conditioning and motivation
Sattva — quality of harmony
Sattvic — of the nature of sattva
Shakti — power, energy, particular of the deepest level, the Goddess
Shiva — divine power of peace and transcendence
Skanda — deity of tejas
Soma — divine nectar or bliss

Srotamsi — channel systems of physical body
Sushumna — central channel or nadi of subtle body

Tamas — quality of darkness and inertia
Tamasic — of the nature of tamas
Tanmatras — sensory potentials or subtle elements (sound, touch, sight, taste, smell)
Tantra — energetic system of working with our higher potentials
Tattvas — cosmic truth principles
Tejas — fire on a vital level

Udana — upward-moving prana
Upaveda — secondary Vedic text

Vata — biological air humor
Vayu — another name for prana or vital force
Vedas — ancient Hindu spiritual system of Self and cosmic knowledge
Vedanga — limb of the Vedas
Vedanta — Self-knowledge aspect of Vedic teaching
Vijnanamaya Kosha — sheath of knowledge or wisdom
Vishnu — divine power of love and protection
Vyana — expansive vital force

Yajna — sacrifice or worship
Yamas — yogic values and principles of social conduct
Yantras — geometric meditation forms
Yoga — science of reintegration with the universal reality

APPENDIX 4

Sanskrit Pronunciation Key

14 Vowels (some have 2 forms)

अ		a	another
आ	ा	ā	father (2 beats)
इ	ि	i	pin
ई	ी	ī	need (2 beats)
उ	ु	u	flute
ऊ	ू	ū	mood (2 beats)
ऋ	ृ	ṛ	macabre
ॠ		ṝ	trill for 2 beats
ऌ		lṛ	table
ए	े	e	etude (2 beats)
ऐ	ै	ai	aisle (2 beats)
ओ	ो	o	yoke (2 beats)
औ	ौ	au	flautist (2 beats)
अं		aṃ	hum
अः		aḥ	out-breath

Eight Intermediate Sounds

य	ya	employable
र	ra	abra cadabra
ल	la	hula
व	va	variety
श	śa	shut
ष	ṣa	shnapps
स	sa	Lisa
ह	ha	honey

25 Consonants

क	ka	paprika
ख	kha	thick honey
ग	ga	saga
‘	gha	big honey
ङ	ṅa	ink
च	ca	chutney
छ	cha	much honey
ज	ja	Japan
झ	jha	raj honey
ञ	ña	inch
ट	ṭa	borscht again
ठ	ṭha	borscht honey
ड	ḍa	shdum
ढ	ḍha	shd hum
ण	ṇa	shnum
त	ta	pasta
थ	tha	eat honey
द	da	soda
ध	dha	good honey
न	na	banana
प	pa	paternal
फ	pha	scoop honey
ब	ba	scuba
भ	bha	rub honey
म	ma	aroma

APPENDIX 5

Bibliography

English

Aurobindo, Sri. LETTERS ON YOGA. Pondicherry, India: Sri Aurobindo Ashram, 1978. Distributed in North America by Lotus Press, www.lotuspress.com

Feuerstein, Georg. The SHAMBHALA ENCYCLOPEDIA OF YOGA. Boston and London: Shambhala Books, 1997.

Feuerstein, Georg. The SHAMBHALA GUIDE TO YOGA. Boston and London: Shambhala Books, 1996.

Feuerstein, Kak and David Frawley. IN SEARCH OF THE CRADLE OF CIVILIZATION. Wheaton, Illinois: Quest Books, 1995.

Frawley, David. ASTROLOGY OF THE SEERS: A GUIDE TO HINDU/ VEDIC ASTROLOGY. Twin Lakes, WI. Lotus Press, 2000.

Frawley, David. AYURVEDA AND THE MIND. Twin Lakes, Wisconsin: Lotus Press, 1997.

Frawley, David. AYURVEDIC HEALING, A COMPREHENSIVE GUIDE. Twin Lakes, WI. Lotus Press, 2000.

Frawley, David. TANTRIC YOGA AND THE WISDOM GODDESSES: SPIRITUAL SECRETS OF AYURVEDA. Twin Lakes, WI. Lotus Press, Second Edition, 2003.

Frawley, David. WISDOM OF THE ANCIENT SEERS: SELECTED MANTRAS FROM THE RIG VEDA. Twin Lakes, WI. Lotus Press, 1992.

Frawley, David and Dr. Vasant Lad. THE YOGA OF HERBS. Twin Lakes, WI. Lotus Press, 1986.

Joshi, Dr. Sunil. AYURVEDA AND PANCHA KARMA. Twin Lakes, Wisconsin: Lotus Press, 1997.

Lad, Dr. Vasant. AYURVEDA, THE SCIENCE OF SELF-HEALING. Twin Lakes, WI. Lotus Press, 1984.

Lad, Dr. Vasant. THE COMPLETE BOOK OF AYURVEDIC HOME REMEDIES. New York City: Harmony Books, 1998.

Morningstar, Amadea. THE AYURVEDIC COOKBOOK. Twin Lakes, Wisconsin: Lotus Press, 1992.

Morningstar, Amadea. AYURVEDIC COOKING FOR WESTERNERS. Twin Lakes, Wisconsin: Lotus Press, 1996.

Niranjananda, Swami. PRANA, PRANAYAMA, PRANA VIDYA. Munger, India: Bihar School of Yoga, 1994.

Shivananda, Swami. PRACTICE OF BRAHMACHARYA. Tehri-Garhwal, India: Divine Life Society, 1988.

Simon, Dr. David. THE WISDOM OF HEALING. New York City, Harmony Books, 1997.

Tarabilda, Ed. AYURVEDA REVOLUTIONIZED. Twin Lakes, Wisconsin: Lotus Press, 1998.

Tierra, Michael. PLANETARY HERBOLOGY. Twin Lakes, WI. Lotus Press, 1988.

Tiwari, Maya. AYURVEDA: LIFE OF BALANCE. Healing Arts Press, 1995.

Yogeshwarananda, Swami. SCIENCE OF THE SOUL. New Delhi, India: Yoga Niketan Trust, 1992.

Yogeshwarananda, Swami. SCIENCE OF PRANA. New Delhi, India: Yoga Niketan Trust, 1992.

Yukteswar, Sri. THE HOLY SCIENCE. Los Angeles, California: Self-Realization Fellowship, 1978.

Sanskrit Texts

ASTANGA HRIDAYA of Vagbhatta.

BHAGAVAD GITA of Sri Krishna.

BRIHAT YOGI YAJNAVALKYA SMRITI.

CARAKA SAMHITA.

Ganapati Muni. RAJA YOGA SUTRAS.

HATHA YOGA PRADIPIKA of Svatmarama.

MAHABHARATA.

SAMKHYA KARIKA of Ishvara Krishna.

SATAPATHA BRAHMANA.

SUSRUTA SAMHITA.

VASISHTA SAMHITA.

188 UPANISHADS.

LAGHU YOGA VASISTHA.

YOGA SUTRAS of Patanjali.

Resources

Vedic Resources Web Site

Note our online books, articles and resources at www.veda net.com covering such topics as Yoga, Ayurveda, Jyotish, Vedanta, Hindu Dharma and ancient history, bridging the entire field of Vedic knowledge.

American Institute of Vedic Studies
Dr. David Frawley (Vamadeva Shastri), Director
PO Box 8357, Santa Fe NM 87504-8357
Ph: 505-983-9385,
Fax: 505-982-5807
Web: www.vedanet.com
Email: vedicinst@aol.com

Aromatherapy Study Programs

Aromatherapy Video and Home Study Program
Michael Scholes (founder of Aroma Vera)
3384 South Robertson Pl.
Los Angeles, CA 90034
Ph: (800)677-2368

Jeanne Rose Aromatherapy and Herbal Healing Intensives
Attn: Jeanne Rose
219 Carl Street
San Francisco, CA 94117

London School of Aromatherapy
P.O. Box 780
London NW5 1DY
England

Pacific Institute of Aromatherapy
Attn: Kurt Schnaubelt
P.O. Box 8723
San Rafael, CA 94903
Ph: (515)479-9121

Quintessence Aromatherapy
Attn: Ann Berwick
P.O. Box 4996
Boulder, CO 80306
Ph: (303)258-3791

Ayurveda Centers and Programs

Australian Institute of Ayurvedic Medicine
19 Bowey Avenue
Enfield S.A. 5085
Australia
Ph: (08)349-7303

Ayurvedic Healing Arts Center
16508 Pine Knoll Road
Grass Valley, CA 95945
Ph: (916)274-9000

Ayurvedic Holistic Center
82A Bayville Ave.
Bayville, NY 11709

The Ayurvedic Institute and Wellness Center

11311 Menaul, NE
Albuquerque, NM 87112
Ph: (505)291-9698
Fax: (505)294-7572

California College of Ayurveda
1117A East Main Street
Grass Valley, CA 95945
Ph: (530)274-9100
Web: www.ayurvedacollege.com
E-Mail: info@ayurvedacollege.com
Training in Ayurveda

Center for Mind, Body Medicine
P.O. Box 1048
La Jolla, CA 92038
Ph: (619)794-2425

The Chopra Center
Deepak Chopra and David Simon
7321 Estrella de Mar Road
Carlsbad, CA 93009
Ph: (888)424-6772
www.chopra.com

Diamond Way Ayurveda
Robert and Melanie Sachs
PO Box 13753
San Luis Obispo, CA 93406
www.diamondwayayurveda.com

John Douillard Life Spa, Rejuvenation through Ayur-Veda
3065 Center Green Dr.
Boulder CO 80301
Ph: 303-442-1164
Fax: 303-442-1240

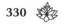

East West College of Herballsm Ayurvedic Program
Represents courses of Dr. David Frawley and Dr. Michael Tierra in UK
Hartswood, Marsh Green, Hartsfield,
E.Sussex TN7 4ET
United Kingdom
Ph: 01342-822312
Fax: 01342-826346
ewcolherb@aol.com

EverGreen Herb Garden and Learning Center, Candis Cantin Packard
PO Box 1445,
Placerville, CA 95667 Ph. & Fax: 530-626-9288
Email: evrgreen@innercite.com

Himalayan Institute
RRI, Box 400
Honesdale, PA 18431
Ph: (800)822-4547

Inside Ayurveda
Bi-monthly, independent publication for ayurvedic professionals
Niika Quistgard
PO Box 3021, Quincy CA 995971-3021
Ph: 530-283-3717
Email: oflife@inreach.com

Institute for Wholistic: Education
3425 Patzke Lane
Racine, WI 53405
Ph: (262)619-1798
Beginner and Advanced Correspondence Courses in Ayurveda
www.wholisticinstitute.org

Integrated Health Systems
3855 Via Nova Marie,
#302 D
Carmel, CA 93923
Ph: (408)476-5130

International Academy of Ayurved
NandNandan, Atreya
Rugnalaya
M.Y. Lele Chowk
Erandawana, Pune:
411 004, India
Ph/Fax:91 212 378532/ 524427
E-Mail: avilele@hotmail.com

International Ayurvedic Institute
111 Elm Street
Suite 103-105
Worcester. MA01609
Ph (508)755-3744
Fax (508)770-0618
E-Mail
ayurveda@hotmail.com

International Federation of Ayurveda
Dr. Krishna Kumar
27 Blight Street
Ridleyton S.A. 5008
Australia
Ph: (08)346-0631

Life Impressions Institute
Attn: Donald VanHowten, Director
613 Kathryn Street Santa Fe, NM 87501
Ph: (505)988-2627

Lotus Ayurvedic Center
4145 Clares St., Suite D
Capitola, CA 95010
Ph: (408)479-1667

Maharishi Ayurved at the Raj
1734 Jasmine Avenue
Fairfield,IA 52556
Ph (800)248-9050
Fax (515)472-2496

Maharishi Health Center
Hale Clinic
7 Park Crescent
London, W14 3H3
England

Natural Therapeutics Center
'Surya Daya'
Gisingham, Nr. Iye
Suffolk, England

New England Institute of Ayurvedic Medicine
111 N. Elm Street
Suites 103-105
Worcester, MA 01609
Ph: (508)755-3744
Fax: (508)770-0618
E-Mail:
ayurveda@hotmail.com

European Institute of Vedic Studies
Atreya Smith, Director
Editions Turiya
I.E.E.V. Sarl, B.P. 4
30170 Monoblet, France
T: 0033 (0) 466 53 7687
F: 0033 (0) 466 53 7688
Email: atreya@free.fr
www.ayurvedicnutrition.com
Ayurvedic Training in Europe.

Victoria Stern, N.D.
P.O. Box 1814
Laguna Beach, CA 92652
Ph: (949)494-8858

Vinayak Ayurveda Center
2509 Virginia NE, Suite D
Albuquerque, NM 87110
Ph: (505)296-6522
Fax: (505)298-2932
Internet: www.ayur.com

Wise Earth School of Ayurveda
Attn: Bri. Maya Tiwari
70 Canter Field Lane
Candler, NC 28715
Ph: (828)258-9999
Teachers and Practitioners
Training Programs Only.

Ayurvedic Cosmetic Companies

Auroma Int'l
PO Box 1008, Dept. YA
Silver Lake, WI 53170
Ph: (262)889-8569
fax: (262) 889 8591
Importer and master
distributor of Auroshikha
Incense, Chandrika
Ayurvedic Soap and Herbal
Vedic Ayurvedic products.
www.auromaintl.com

Bindi Facial Skin Care
A Division of Pratima Inc.
109-17 72nd Road
Lower Level
Forest Hills, New York
11375
Ph: (718)268-7348

Devi Inc. (for Shivani
product line)
Attn: Anjali Mahaldar
P.O. Box 377
Lancaster, MA 01523
Ph: (800)237-8221
Fax: (508)368-0455

Gajee Herbals
The Khenpo Company
Attn: Gayatri Puri, Owner
17595 Harvard Street,
C531
Irvine, CA 92714
Ph: (714)250-6027

Internatural
PO Box 489, Dept. YA
Twin Lakes, WI 53181 USA
800 643 4221 (toll free
order line)
262 889 8581 (office
phone)
262 889 8591 (fax)
email: internatural@
lotuspress.com
web site:
www.internatural.com
Retail mail order and
internet reseller of essential
oils, herbs, spices,
supplements, herbal
remedies, incense, books
and other supplies.

Lotus Brands, Inc.
PO Box 325, Dept. YA
Twin Lakes, WI 53181
Ph: (262)889-8561
Fax: (262)889-8591
lotusbrands@lotuspress.com
www.lotusbrands.com
Manufacturer and
distributor of natural
personal care and herbal
products, massage oils,
essential oils, incense and
aromatherapy items.

Lotus Light Enterprises
PO Box 1008, Dept. YA
Silver Lake, WI 53170 USA
800 548 3824 (toll free
order line)

262 889 8501 (office
phone)
262 889 8591 (fax)
lotuslight@lotuspress.com
www.lotuslight.com
Wholesale distributor of
essential oils, herbs, spices,
supplements, herbal
remedies, incense, books
and other supplies. Must
supply resale certificate
number or practitioner
license to obtain catalog of
more than 10,000 items.

Siddhi Ayurvedic Beauty Products
C/O Vinayak Ayurveda
Center
2509 Virginia NE, Suite D
Albuquerque, NM 87110
Ph: (505)296-6522
Fax: (505)298-2932

Swami Sada Shiva Tirtha Ayurvedic Holistic Center
82A Bayville Avenue
Bayville, NY 11709
Ph/Fax: (516)628-8200

TEJ Beauty Enterprises, Inc.
(an Ayurvedic Beauty
Salon)
162 West 56th St., Rm 201
New York, NY 10019
(owner: Pratima Raichur,
founder of Bindi)
Ph: (212)581-8136

Ayurvedic Herbal Suppliers

Auroma Int'l
PO Box 1008, Dept. YA
Silver Lake, WI 53170

Ph: (262)889-8569
fax: (262) 889 8591
www.auromaintl.com
Importer and master
distributor of Auroshikha
Incense, Chandrika
Ayurvedic Soap and Herbal
Vedic Ayurvedic products.

Ayur Herbal Corporation
PO Box 6390, Dept. YA
Santa Fe, NM 87502
Ph: (262)889-8569
www.herbalvedic.com

Ayush Herbs, Inc.
10025 N.E. 4th Street
Bellevue, WA 98004
Ph: (800)925-1371

**Bazaar of India
Imports, Inc.**
1810 University Avenue
Berkeley, CA 94703
Ph: (800)261-7662;
(510)548-4110

Diamond Way Ayurveda
Robert and Melanie Sachs
PO Box 13753
San Luis Obispo, CA 93406
805-543-9291
www.diamondwayayurveda.com

**Dr. Singha's Mustard Bath
and More**
Attn: Anna Searles
Natural Therapeutic Centre
2500 Side Cove
Austin, TX 78704
Ph: (800)856-2862

Bio Veda
215 North Route 303
Congers, NY 10920-1726
Ph: (800)292-6002

Frontier Herbs
P.O. Box 229
Norway, IA 52318
Ph: (800)669-3275

HerbalVedic Products
P.O. Box 6390
Santa Fe, NM 87502
www.herbalvedic.com

Internatural
PO Box 489, Dept. YA
Twin Lakes, WI 53181 USA
800 643 4221 (toll free
order line)
262 889 8581 (office
phone)
262 889 8591 (fax)
email: internatural@
lotuspress.com
web site:
www.internatural.com
Retail mail order and
internet reseller of essential
oils, herbs, spices,
supplements, herbal
remedies, incense, books
and other supplies.

Kanak
P.O. Box 13653
Albuquerque, NM
87192-3653
Ph: (505)275-2469

Lotus Brands, Inc.
PO Box 325, Dept. YA
Twin Lakes, WI 53181
Ph: (262)889-8561
Fax: (262)889-8591
www.lotusbrands.com

Lotus Herbs
1505 42nd Ave., Suite 19
Capitola, CA 95010
Ph: (408)479-1667

Lotus Light Enterprises
PO Box 1008, Dept. YA
Silver Lake, WI 53170 USA
800 548 3824 (toll free
order line)
262 889 8501 (office)
262 889 8591 (fax)
lotuslight@lotuspress.com
www.lotuslight.com
Wholesale distributor of
essential oils, herbs, spices,
supplements, herbal
remedies, incense, books
and other supplies. must
supply resale certificate
number or practitioner
license to obtain catalog of
more than 10,000 items.

**Maharishi Ayurveda
Products International**
417 Bolton Road,
P.O. Box 541
Lancaster, MA 01523
Info: (800)843-8332 x903
Order: (800)255-8332
x 903

Quantum Publication, Inc.
P.O. Box 1088
Sudbury, MA 01776
Ph: (800)858-1808

**Vinayak Panchakarma
Chikitsalaya**
Y.M.C.A Complex,
Situbuldi
Nagpur (Maharastra State)
India 440 012
Ph: 011-91-712-538983
Fax: 011-91-712-552409
Retail/Wholesale

Yoga of Life Center
2726 Tramway N.E.
Albuquerque, NM 87122
Ph: (505)275-6141

Bodywork Training

The Center For Release and Integration
450 Hillside Drive
Mill Valley, CA 94941

Dr. Jay Scherer's Academy of Natural Healing
1443 St. Francis Drive
Santa Fe, NM 87505

The Rolf Institute
205 Canyon Blvd.
Boulder, CO 80302

The Upledger Institute
1211 Prosperity Farms Rd.
Palm Beach Gardens, FL 33410

The Feldenkrais Guild
524 Ellsworth St. SW
P.O. Box 489
Albany, OR 97321

Correspondence Courses

American Institute of Vedic Studies
Dr. David Frawley, Director
P.O. Box 8357
Santa Fe, NM 87504-8357
Ph: (505)983-9385
Fax: (505)982-5807
E-Mail: vedicinst@aol.com
Web: www.vedanet.com
Correspondence courses in Ayurveda and Vedic Astrology.

Lessons and Lectures in Ayur-veda by Dr. Robert Svoboda
P.O. Box 23445
Albuquerque, NM 87192-1445
Ph: (505)291-9698

Institute for Wholistic Education
3425 Patzke Lane
Racine, WI 53405
Ph: (262)619-1798
www.wholisticinstitute.org

Beauty and Quality Ayurvedic Supplements

Auroma Int'l
PO Box 1008
Dept. YA
Silver Lake, WI 53170
Ph: (262) 889-8569
Fax: (262) 889-8591
Importer and master distributor Auroshikha Incense, Chandrika Ayurvedic Soap and Herbal Vedic Ayurvedic products.
www.auromaintl.com

Ayur Herbal Corporation
P.O. Box 6390 YA
Santa Fe, NM 87502
Ph: (262)889-8569
fax: (262) 889-8591
Manufacturer of Herbal Vedic Ayurvedic products.
www.herbalvedic.com

Internatural
P.O. Box 489, Dept. YA
Twin Lakes,W1 53181 USA
800 643 4221
(toll free order line)
262 889 8581(office)
262 889 8591 (fax)
email:
internatural@lotuspress.com
website:
www.internatural.com
Retail mail order and internet reseller of essential oils, herbs, spices, supplements, herbal remedies, incense, books and other supplies.

Lotus Brands, Inc.
P.O. Box 325, Dept. YA
Twin Lakes, W1 53181 Ph: (262)889-8561
Fax: (262)889-8591
email:
lotusbrands@lotuspress.com
website:
www.lotusbrands.com Man ufacturer and distributor of natural personal care and herbal products, massage oils, essential oils, incense and aromatherapy items.

Lotus Light Enterprises
P.O. Box 1008 Dept. YA
Silver Lake, WI 53170 USA
800 548 3824 (toll free order line)
262 889 8501(office)
262 889 8591 (fax)
email:
lotuslight@lotuspress.com
website: www.lotuslight.com
Wholesale distributor of essential oils, herbs, spices, supplements, herbal remedies, incense, books and other supplies. Must supply resale certificate number or practitioner license to obtain catalog of more than 10,000 items.

Maharishi Ayur-Veda
Products International
417 Bolton Road
P.O. Box 54
Lancaster, MA 01523
Ph: (800)ALL-VEDA
Fax: (508)368-7475

New Moon Extracts
P.O. Box 1947
Brattleborough, VT
05302-1947
Ph: (800)543-7279

Spectrum Natural Omega
3 Oil - The Oil Company
133 Copeland Street
Petaluma, CA 94952

Universal Light, Inc.
PO Box 261, Dept. YA
Wilmot, WI 53192
Ph: 262 889 8571
Fax: 262 889 8591
Importer and Master
Distributor for Vicco
Herbal Toothpaste.

Color, Sound, and Gems

PAZ
P.O. Box 4859
Albuquerque, NM 87196
For open-backed gemstone
settings.

Color Therapy Eyewear
C/O Terri Perrigone-Messer
P.O. Box 3114
Diamond Springs, CA
95619

Lumatron (light device)
C/O Ernie Baker
515 Pierce Street #3
San Francisco, CA 94117
Ph: (415)626-0083

Genesis (sound device)
Medical Massage Therapy
Attn: Tina Shinn
1857 Northwest Blvd.
Annex
Columbus, Ohio 43212
Ph: (614)488-5244

Essential Oil Supplies

Aromatherapy Supply
Unit W3
The Knoll Business Center
Old Shoreham Road
Hove, Sussex BN3 7GS
England

Aroma Vera
3384 South Robertson Pl.
Los Angeles, CA 90034
Ph: (800)669-9514

Auroma Int'l
PO Box 1008, Dept. YA
Silver Lake, WI 53170
Ph: (262)889-8569
Fax: (262) 889 8591
Importer and master
distributor of Auroshikha
Incense, Chandrika
Ayurvedic Soap and Herbal
Vedic Ayurvedic products.
www.auromaintl.com

Fenmail Tisserand Oils
P.O. Box 48
Spalding, LINCS PE11 ADS
England

Internatural
PO Box 489, Dept. YA
Twin Lakes, WI 53181 USA
800 643 4221 (toll free
order line)
262 889 8581 (office
phone)

262 889 8591 (fax)
email: internatural@
lotuspress.com
web site:
www.internatural.com
Retail mail order and
internet reseller of essential
oils, herbs, spices,
supplements, herbal
remedies, incense, books
and other supplies.

Lotus Brands, Inc.
PO Box 325, Dept. YA
Twin Lakes, WI 53181
Ph: (262)889-8561
Fax: (262)889-8591
email: lotusbrands@
lotuspress.com
web site:
www.lotusbrands.com
Manufacturer and
distributor of natural
personal care and herbal
products, massage oils,
essential oils, incense and
aromatherapy items.

Lotus Light Enterprises
PO Box 1008, Dept. YA
Silver Lake, WI 53170 USA
800 548 3824 (toll free
order line)
262 889 8501 (office
phone)
262 889 8591 (fax)
email:
lotuslight@lotuspress.com
web site:
www.lotuslight.com
Wholesale distributor of
essential oils, herbs, spices,
supplements, herbal
remedies, incense, books
and other supplies. Must
supply resale certificate
number or practitioner

license to obtain catalog of more than 10,000 items.

Private Universe
P.O. Box 3122
Winter Park, FL 32790
Ph: (407)644-7203

Oshadi Ayus - Quality Life Products
15, Monarch Bay Plaza
Suite 346
Monarch Beach, CA 92629
Ph: (800)947-1008
Fax; (714)240-1104

Primavera
D 8961 Sulzberg
Germany
08376-808-0

Original Swiss Aromatics
P.O. Box 606
San Rafael, CA 94915
Ph: (415)459-3998

Exercise Programs and Information

Callanetic Headquarters
1700 Broadway
Suite 2000
Denver, CO 80290
Ph: (303)831-4455

Vega Study Center
1511 Robinson Street
Oroville, CA 95965
Ph: (916)533-7702
For Sotai instructions - books.

Satori Resources
732 Hamlin Way
San Leandro, CA 94578
For Tai Chi Chih.

Kushi Institute
P.O. Box 7
Becket, MA 01223
Ph: (413)623-5741
For Do-in.

Natural Ingredients

Aloe Farms
Box 125
Los Fresnos, TX 78566
Ph: (800)262-6771
For aloe vera juice, gel, powder and capsules.

Arya Laya Skin Care Center
Rolling Hills Estates, CA 90274
For carrot oil.

Aubrey Organics
4419 North Manhattan Ave
Tampa, FL 33614
For rosa mosquita oil and a large variety of natural cosmetics and shampoos.

Body Shop
45 Horsehill Road
Cedar Knolls, NJ 07927-2014
Ph: (800)541-2535
Aloe vera, nut and seed oils, cosmetics, make-up, brushes, loofahs and much more.

Culpepper Ltd.
21 Bruton Street
London W1X 7DA
England
Variety of natural seed, nut, and kernal oils, essential oils, herbs, books and cosmetics.

Desert Whale Jojoba Co.
P.O. Box 41594
Tucson, AZ 85717
Ph: (602)882-4195
For jojoba products and many other natural oils, including rice bran, pecan, macadamia nut and apricot kernal.

Everybody Ltd.
1738 Pearl Street
Boulder, CO 80302
Ph: (800)748-5675
Large variety of oils, oil blends and cosmetics.

Flora Inc.
P.O. Box 950
805 East Badger Road
Lynden, WA 98264
Ph: (800)446-2110
For flax seed oil, herbal supplements for skin, hair, nails and cosmetics.

Green Earth Farm
P.O. Box 672
65 1/2 North 8th Street
Saguache, CO 81149
For calendula oil, creme, and herbal bath.

The Heritage Store, Inc.
P.O. Box 444
Virginia Beach, VA 23458
Ph: (804)428-0100
Castor oil, organic ghee,
cocoa butter, massage oils,
flower-waters, essential
oils, cosmetics and natural
home remedies.

Internatural
PO Box 489, Dept. YA
Twin Lakes, WI 53181 USA
800 643 4221 (toll free
order line)
262 889 8581 (office
phone)
262 889 8591 (fax)
email:
internatural@lotuspress.com
web site:
www.internatural.com
Retail mail order and
internet reseller of essential
oils, herbs, spices,
supplements, herbal
remedies, incense, books
and other supplies.

**Janca's Jojoba Oil and
Seed Company**
456 E. Juanita #7
Mesa, AZ 85204
Ph: (602)497-9494
(jojoba oil, butter, wax,
and seeds. Also a large
variety of naturally pressed
unusual oils, such as
camellia, kukui nut, and
grapeseed. Also have clay,
aloe products, essential
oils, and their own line of
cosmetics)

Lotus Brands, Inc.
PO Box 325, Dept. YA
Twin Lakes, WI 53181
Ph: (262)889-8561
Fax: (262)889-8591
email:
lotusbrands@lotuspress.com
web site:
www.lotusbrands.com
Manufacturer and
distributor of natural
personal care and herbal
products, massage oils,
essential oils, incense and
aromatherapy items.

Lotus Light Enterprises
PO Box 1008, Dept. YA
Silver Lake, WI 53170 USA
800 548 3824 (toll free
order line)
262 889 8501 (office
phone)
262 889 8591 (fax)
email:
lotuslight@lotuspress.com
web site:
www.lotuslight.com
Wholesale distributor of
essential oils, herbs,
spices, supplements,
herbal remedies, incense,
books and other supplies.
must supply resale
certificate number or
practitioner license to
obtain catalog of more
than 10,000 items.

Weleda, Inc.
841 South Main Street
Spring Valley, NY 10977
For calendula oil and a
large variety of natural
cosmetics.

Non-Denominational Meditation Training

Shambhala Training
International Executive
Offices
1084 Tower Road
Halifax, Nova Scotia
Canada B3H 265

Organic Milk/ Certified Raw Milk Suppliers

Alta Delta Certified
Raw Milk
P.O. Box 388
City of Industry, CA 91747
Ph: (818)964-6401
(non pasteurized, non-
homogenized milk)

Natural Horizons, Inc.
7490 Clubhouse Road
Boulder, CO 80301
Ph: (303)530-2711
(organic/pasteurized, non-
homogenized milk; whole,
low-fat, skim buttermilk
and cream)

Organic Valley Family
of Farms
C/O Cropp Cooperative
La Farge, WI 54639
Ph: (608)625-2602
Organic butter, non-
homogenized low-fat milk.

Pancha Karma Kitchen Equipment

Earth Fare
Attn: Roger Derrough
66 Westgate Parkway
Asheville, NC 28806
Ph: (704)253-7656
Carries hand grinders and suribachi clay pots and bowls.

Garber Hardware
49 Eighth Avenue
New York, NY 10014
Carries hand grinders, but no mail order.

Sesam Muhle Natural Products
RR1
Durham, Ontario
Canada, NOG 1RO
Ph: (519)369-6326
Carries a line of hand grinders and flakers for grains and legumes, made in Germany.

Taj Mahal Imports
1594 Woodcliff Drive, N.E.
Atlanta, GA 30329
Ph: (404)321-5940
Carries a full line of Indian kitchen equipment.

To Receive Pancha Karma

Diamond Way Health Associates
214 Girard Blvd., NE
Albuquerque, NM 87106
Ph: (505)265-4826

Dr. Lobsang Rapgay
2206 Benecia Ave.
Wetwood, CA 90064

Spa Medicine

Ancient Way Ayurvedic Health Spa
Attn: Dr. Dennis Thompson
3260 47th St., #205A
Boulder, CO 80301
E-Mail:
drtdrt@concentric.net

Vedic Astrology

American Council of Vedic Astrology (ACVA)
P.O. Box 2149
Sedona, AZ 86339
Ph: (800)900-6595;
(520)282-6595
Fax: (520)282-6097
Web:
www.vedicastrology.org
E-Mail: acva@sedona.net
Conferences, tutorial and training programs.

American Institute of Vedic Studies
Dr. David Frawley, Director
P.O. Box 8357
Santa Fe, NM 87504-8357
Ph: (505)983-9385
Fax: (505)982-5807
E-Mail:
vedicinst@aol.com
Web: www.vedanet.com
Correspondence courses in Ayurveda and Vedic Astrology.

Videos

Feldenkrais Resources
Ph: (800)765-1907

Wishing Well Video
P.O. Box 1008
Dept. YA
Silver Lake, WI 53170 USA
Ph: (262)889-8501
(wholesale & retail)

About the Author

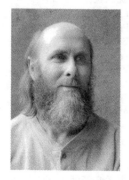

Dr. David Frawley and the American Institute of Vedic Studies

Dr. David Frawley (Vamadeva Shastri) is recognized both in India and the West for his knowledge of Vedic teachings, which include Ayurveda, Vedic Astrology, and Yoga. He is the author of twenty books published over the last twenty years, including Ayurveda and the Mind, Yoga of Herbs, Ayurvedic Healing and Astrology of the Seers. His Vedic translations and historical studies on ancient India have received much acclaim, as have his journalistic works on modern India. Dr. Frawley is the director of the American Institute of Vedic studies and is on the editorial board of the magazine Yoga International for which he is a frequent contributor. He is also the president of the American Council of Vedic Astrology (ACVA).

American Institute of Vedic Studies

The American Institute of Vedic Studies offers programs in Ayurveda, Vedic astrology and related Vedic disciplines, including research into the Vedas and their historical and spiritual background. The Institute is affiliated with various organizations including the California College of Ayurveda, the New England Institute of Ayurvedic Medicine, the East West College of Herbalism (UK), the American Council of Vedic Astrology (ACVA), and the World Association of Vedic Studies (WAVES). It works with different Hindu groups and national organizations in India to promote the cause of Vedic education.

Ayurvedic Medicine Correspondence Course

This comprehensive practical program covers all the main aspects of Ayurvedic theory, diagnosis and practice, with a special emphasis on herbal medicine using both Eastern and Western herbs. It sets forth the system of Ayurvedic anatomy and physiology, differential diagnosis of disease and constitutional treatment methods. It goes in detail into Yoga philosophy and Ayurvedic psychology, showing an integral approach of mind-body medicine. The course is designed for Health Care Professionals as well as serious students to provide the foundation for becoming an Ayurvedic practitioner.

The course of over six hundred pages comes in four sections and has recently been revised and expanded. Certification is given to students who answer all test questions satisfactorily, and credit for 250 hours of study in Ayurveda, as well as options for further study both in India and the United States. Since 1988 over two thousand people from all over the world have taken it.

Vedic Astrology Correspondence Course

This comprehensive home study course explains Vedic astrology in clear and modern terms, providing many practical insights how to use and adapt the system. For those who have difficulty approaching the Vedic system, the course provides many keys for unlocking its language and its methodology for the Western student. It covers planets, signs, houses, aspects, yogas, nakshatras, dashas, ashtakavarga, and more, with a special emphasis on gem therapy and medical astrology.

The goal of the course is to provide the foundation for the student to become a professional Vedic astrologer. The orientation of the course is twofold: To teach the language and way of thinking of Vedic Astrology, and to set forth the Astrology of Healing (Ayurvedic Astrology).

The course of over six hundred pages comes in four sections, which includes one workbook that has been recently added. Certification is given to students who answer all test questions satisfactorily and credit for 200 hours of study in Vedic astrology. The course can be taken as part of a longer 600-hour tutorial program through the American Council of Vedic Astrology (ACVA). The course starts at a beginning level but goes into depth into its subject. Since 1986 over two thousand people have taken it.

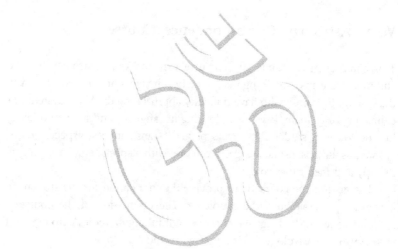

Index

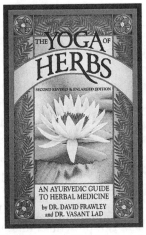

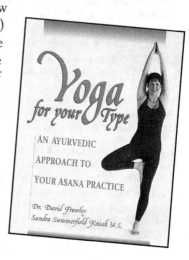

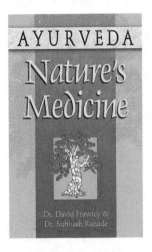

AYURVEDA AND THE MIND

The Healing of Consciousness

DR. DAVID FRAWLEY

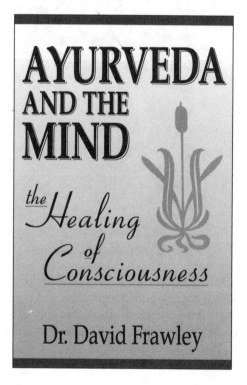

"*Ayurveda and the Mind* addresses, with both sensitivity and lucidity, how to create wholeness in Body, Mind and Spirit. This book opens the door to a new energetic psychology that provides practical tools to integrate the many layers of life. Dr. Frawley has added another important volume to his many insightful books on Ayurveda and Vedic sciences."

DEEPAK CHOPRA M.D.

AUTHOR, *Ageless Body, Timeless Mind*